More Praise for <u>The Instinct to Heal</u>:

"Offers a roundup of effective techniques—some cutting edge, some tried-and-true—for treating depression without drugs or talk therapy."

—READER'S DIGEST (EDITOR'S CHOICE)

"*The Instinct to Heal* will help anyone expand their concepts of health and health care to a more majestic level."

—LARRY DOSSEY, M.D., BESTSELLING AUTHOR OF *HEALING BEYOND THE BODY, REINVENTING MEDICINE,* AND *HEALING WORDS*

"David Servan-Schreiber has an intriguing explanation for the emotional woes plaguing America today. . . . Seeing real people put it to work makes the book worth reading—and may help you tap into your own 'instinct to heal.'"

—*ALTERNATIVE HEALING*

"The scientist and physician David Servan-Schreiber has provided a wonderful manual to help reconcile our emotional and rational brains . . . [he] bases his advice about how to improve our lives on a profound understanding of how the human brain works, on a broad synthesis of the latest knowledge in neuropsychology, as well as his own clinical and research experience. The book is deeply satisfying intellectually, yet crystal-clear and user-friendly."

—MIHALY CSIKSZENTMIHALYI, PH.D., BESTSELLING AUTHOR OF *FLOW, BEING ADOLESCENT, THE EVOLVING SELF,* AND *CREATIVITY*

"This is a fascinating journey into the relationships between our various biological and emotional systems that shows we have an instinctual ability to heal ourselves. This is a definitive work on new research in the relationship between the mind and body and a recommended read."

—*THE MIDWEST BOOK REVIEW*

"Servan-Schreiber, himself a first-rate scientist, only discusses approaches that he feels have been studied sufficiently by rigorous scientific methods to make him a believer. I learned a lot."

—JOSEPH LEDOUX, PH.D., THE HENRY AND LUCY MOSES PROFESSOR OF SCIENCE AT NYU AND AUTHOR OF *THE EMOTIONAL BRAIN* AND *SYNAPTIC SELF*

The
INSTINCT
to
HEAL

The
INSTINCT
to
HEAL

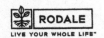
RODALE
LIVE YOUR WHOLE LIFE™
Every day our brands connect with and inspire millions of people to live a life of the mind, body, spirit — a whole life.

This book was originally published in French, as *Guérir le stress, l'anxiété et la dépression sans médicaments ni pyschanalyse*, by Editions Robert Laffont, S.A., Paris, 2003.

© 2003, 2004 by David Servan-Schreiber

Printed in the United States of America
Rodale Inc. makes every effort to use acid-free ∞, recycled paper ♲.

Illustrations on pages 39 and 57 reprinted courtesy of Editions Robert Laffont, S. A., Paris.
Book design by Mark McGarry, Texas Type & Book Works
Library of Congress Cataloging-in-Publication Data

Servan-Schreiber, David.
    [Guérir le stress, l'anxiété et la dépression sans médicaments ni psychanalyse. English]
    The instinct to heal : curing stress, anxiety, and depression without drugs and and without talk therapy / by David Servan-Schreiber.
        p.   cm.
    Includes index.
    Originally published in French.
    ISBN-13 978–1–57954–902–2 hardcover
    ISBN-10 1–57954–902–0 hardcover
    ISBN-13 978–1–59486–158–1 paperback
    ISBN-10 1–59486–158–7 paperback
    1. Depression, Mental—Alternative treatment.   2. Anxiety—Alternative treatment.   I. Title.
    RC537.S47513   2004
    616.85'2706—dc22   2003022471

Distributed to the trade by Holtzbrinck Publishers
    4   6   8   10   9   7   5   3   hardcover
 12 14 16 18 20 19 17 15 13 11   paperback

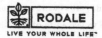

Dedication

To the residents of Presbyterian-Shadyside Hospital of the University of Pittsburgh.

In order to be worthy of teaching them, I have had to relearn everything I thought I knew. Through them, I wish to dedicate this book to all physicians and therapists, everywhere in the world, who burn with curiosity about human beings and with a passion to heal.

Table of Contents

Caveats 1

1 A New Emotion Medicine 3

2 Discontent in Neurobiology:
  The Difficult Marriage of Two Brains 13

3 The Heart and Its Reasons 33

4 Living with Heart Coherence 51

5 Eye Movement Desensitization and Reprocessing
  (EMDR): The Mind's Own Healing Mechanism 69

6 EMDR in Action 85

7 The Energy of Light:
  Resetting Your Biological Clock 99

8 The Power of Qi:
  Acupuncture Directly Affects the Emotional Brain . . 109

9 The Revolution in Nutrition:
   Omega-3 Fatty Acids Feed the Emotional Brain ... 123

10 Prozac or Puma? 145

11 Love Is a Biological Need 161

12 Enhancing Emotional Communication 175

13 Listening with the Heart 193

14 The Larger Connection 207

15 Getting Started 215

    Epilogue 231

    Acknowledgments 233

    Resources 239

    Notes 251

    Index 281

Caveats

"Heal" is a powerful word. Isn't it presumptuous for a physician to use such a word in the title of a book on stress, anxiety, and depression? I've thought a lot about this question.

To me, "healing" means that patients are no longer suffering from the symptoms that they complained of when they first consulted, and that these symptoms do not come back after the treatment has been completed. This is what happens when we treat an infection with antibiotics. This is also precisely what I have observed when I started to practice with the methods described in this book, and this is borne out by some of the research studies. In the end, I decided it was alright to use "heal" in the title of the book, because not using it would have been dishonest.

The ideas presented in this book are largely inspired by the works of Antonio Damasio, Daniel Goleman, Tom Lewis, Dean Ornish, Andrew Weil, Judith Hermann, Bessel van der Kolk, Joe LeDoux, Mihaly Csikszentmihalyi, Scott Shannon, and many other physicians

and researchers. Over the years, we have taken part in the same conferences, talked to the same collegues, and read the same scientific
literature. Of course, there are many areas of overlap, common references, and similar ideas in their books and this one. However, coming
after them, I have had the liberty to draw on their talent for exposing
scientific ideas in simple, understandable terms. I wish to thank them
here for all that I borrowed from their works and for any good idea
that this book may contain. Of course, ideas with which they may not
necessarily agree remain my entire responsibility.

All the cases of patients presented in the following pages are
drawn from my own clinical experience, except for a few that were
described in the scientific literature and that are referred to as such.
Naturally, names and all identifying information have been changed
to protect the confidentiality of the patients described. For literary
reasons, I have chosen, in a few instances, to bring together the clinical features of two different patients into a single story.

1

A New Emotion Medicine

Doubting everything and believing everything are two equally convenient solutions that guard us from having to think.

—HENRI POINCARÉ, *OF SCIENCE AND HYPOTHESES*

Every life is unique . . . and every life is difficult. We are often surprised at our own envy toward someone else.

"If only I were beautiful like Marilyn Monroe."

"If only I were a rock star."

"If only I lived the adventures of Ernest Hemingway."

By becoming someone else, we would not have our usual problems—that much is true. But we would have others—theirs!

Marilyn Monroe was perhaps the sexiest, most famous, and most coveted of all women of her generation. Yet, she always felt lonely and she drowned her distress in alcohol. She eventually died of an overdose of barbiturates. Kurt Cobain, the lead singer of the rock band Nirvana, became a superstar over a few years. He killed himself before he reached 30. Hemingway, whose Nobel Prize and extraordinary life did not save him from a deep existential void, also committed suicide. Neither talent, nor glory, power, money, or the admiration of women and men can make the essence of life fundamentally easier.

There are, however, people who seem to live with harmony. Most often they have the feeling that life is generous. They are able to enjoy the people around them and the little pleasures of every day: meals, sleep, projects, relationships. They do not belong to a cult or a specific religion. They do not live in a particular country. Some are rich, others are not. Some are married, others live alone. Some have special talents, others are quite ordinary. They have all experienced failures, disappointments, dark moments. Nobody escapes from hardships. But on the whole, these people seem better equipped to overcome obstacles. They seem to have a special ability to get through misfortune, to give meaning to their lives, as if they had a closer relationship with themselves, with others, and with what they have chosen to do with their existence.

How does one become so resilient? How can we build a propensity toward happiness? I spent 20 years studying and practicing medicine, mainly in major universities of the United States, Canada, and France, but also with Tibetan doctors and Native American shamans. Over that time, I found certain keys that turned out to be useful for my patients as well as myself. To my surprise, these were not the methods I'd learned at the university. They involved neither drugs nor the usual talk therapies.

The Turning Point

I did not come to this conclusion—and this new style of medicine— easily. I started my career in medicine as a purebred scientist. After graduating from medical school, I left medicine for five years in order to study how neurons arrange themselves in networks to produce thoughts and emotions. I did a Ph.D. in cognitive neuroscience at Carnegie Mellon University under the supervision of Herbert Simon, Ph.D., one of the handful of psychologists ever awarded a Nobel Prize, and of James McClelland, Ph.D., one of the founders of modern neural network theory. The main result of my thesis was published in the journal *Science*, a prestigious publication in which every scientist hopes to see his work appear one day.

After this training in hard sciences, it was actually difficult for me to return to the clinical world and to complete my residency in psychiatry. Working with patients seemed too "soft," too vague, almost . . . too easy. Clinical work had very little in common with the hard data and mathematical precision that I had become accustomed to. However, I reassured myself that I was learning how to treat psychiatric patients in one of the most hard-nosed and research-oriented departments of psychiatry in the country. At the University of Pittsburgh, it was said that psychiatry received more federal research funding than any other department in the school of medicine, including the prestigious department of transplant surgery. With a certain hubris, we thought of ourselves as "clinical scientists."

Shortly after that, I was awarded enough grants from the National Institutes of Health and from private foundations to start my own laboratory. Things could not have looked more promising and my curiosity for new knowledge, and for solid facts, promised to be fed. However, in short order, a few experiences would change my view of medicine completely, and also change the course of my career.

One was a trip to India, for the medical relief group Doctors Without Borders/Médecins Sans Frontières, for whom I worked as a member of the United States board of directors from 1991 to 2000. I was going to India to work with Tibetan refugees in Dharamsala, the home base of the Dalai Lama. There, I observed a traditional Tibetan medicine in which practitioners diagnosed diseases and "imbalances" through lengthy palpation of the pulses of both wrists and inspection of the tongue and urine. These practitioners treated only with acupuncture, traditional herbs, and the instruction to meditate. They seemed every bit as successful with a variety of patients suffering from chronic illnesses as we were in the West, yet their treatments had remarkably fewer side effects and cost a lot less.

As a psychiatrist, most of my own patients were suffering from chronic diseases. (Depression, anxiety, bipolar disorder, and stress are all chronic conditions.) I started to wonder about whether the contempt for traditional approaches I had been taught throughout my training was based on objective facts or on ignorance. Indeed, if the track record of Western medicine was outstanding for acute conditions such as pneumonia, appendicitis, or bone fractures, it was far from stellar for most chronic conditions, including anxiety and depression.

The other challenge to my own medical arrogance was a more personal experience. During a visit to France a very close childhood friend told me about her recovery from a serious depression. She had refused the medications that her doctor had offered and she had sought the care of a sort of healer. She was treated with "sophrology," a technique that involves deep relaxation and reexperiencing of old, buried emotions. She had come out of this treatment "better than normal." Not only was she no longer depressed, she was also freed from the weight of 30 years of unexpressed grief over the loss of her father, who had died when she was 6 years old.

My friend had found a new energy, a new lightness and clarity of purpose that had never been a part of who she was before the treatment. I was happy for her but also shocked and disappointed in myself. In all my years of studying the mind and the brain, in all the training I had received both in scientific psychology and then in psychiatry, I had never witnessed such profound results, nor been shown such treatment methods. In fact, I had been actively discouraged from looking into them—as if they were the purview of charlatans, not worthy of medical doctors and not even worthy of scientific curiosity.

Yet, my friend had achieved far more than I had learned to expect from the techniques I had been taught: psychiatric medications and conventional talk therapy.

If she had come to *me* as her psychiatrist, I would most likely have limited her chances of finding the growth that she had experienced through the unusual treatment she had chosen. If, after all these years of training, I couldn't have helped someone I really cared about, what was all my knowledge really worth? In the months and years that followed, I learned to open my mind—and my heart—to different and often more effective ways of healing others.

The seven natural treatment approaches that I will describe in this book all capitalize on the mind and brain's own healing mechanisms for recovering from depression, anxiety, and stress. All seven methods have been researched and studies documenting their benefits have been published in prestigious scientific journals. Because the mechanisms through which they operate remain poorly understood, these methods have remained largely excluded from the mainstream of medicine and psychiatry. Conventional medicine should, legitimately, seek an understanding of how treatments actually work. However, it is not legitimate to exclude treatments that have been shown to work and to be safe simply because we do not understand *how* they work. Today, the demand is so great for such approaches that it will no longer be possible to set them aside. And there are good reasons for a more open approach.

The Sad State of Affairs

Disorders linked to stress—including depression and anxiety—are widespread in our societies. The numbers are alarming: Clinical studies suggest that 50 to 75 percent of all visits to the doctor are primarily related to stress, and that, in terms of mortality, stress poses a more serious risk factor than tobacco.[1,2] In fact, eight out of ten of the most commonly used medications in the United States are intended to treat problems directly related to stress: antidepressants, anxiolytics and sleeping pills, antacids for heartburn and ulcers, and medications for high blood pressure.[3] In 1999, three of the top-selling drugs of any sort in the United States were three antidepressants (Prozac, Paxil, and Zoloft).[4] In fact, it is estimated that about one in eight Americans has taken an antidepressant, almost half of them for more than a year.[5]

Even though stress, anxiety, and depression are on the increase, those who suffer from these problems are suspicious of the two traditional pillars of emotional treatment: talk therapy and medications. Already in 1997, a Harvard study showed, a *majority* of Americans suffering from these conditions preferred "alternative and complementary" methods over traditional psychotherapies or drugs.[6]

Psychoanalysis is losing ground. Having dominated psychiatry for 30 years, its credibility is dwindling because its effectiveness hasn't been sufficiently proven.[7] If we live in New York, one of the few remaining bastions of psychoanalysis in the English-speaking world, we may all know someone who greatly benefited from analytic treatment, but we also know a lot of other people who have been going in circles on the analyst's couch for years.

Today, the most common form of psychotherapy is cognitive-behavior therapy. It has a remarkable track record, with a wealth of studies showing its effectiveness in conditions as varied as depression and obsessive-compulsive disorder. Patients who have learned to control their thoughts and to systematically examine their assumptions and beliefs clearly do better than those who haven't. However, many patients feel that the often exclusive focus on present thoughts and behaviors fails to encompass the whole dimension of their lives—including, most importantly, their body.

Other than psychotherapy, there is "biological psychiatry." This is the modern form of psychiatry that primarily treats patients with psychotropic medications like Prozac, Zoloft, Paxil, Xanax, lithium, Zyprexa, etcetera. In the trenches of daily medical practice, psychotropic medications dominate the field almost completely. Talk therapy—though proven effective—is used much more rarely. The prescription reflex has become so common that if a patient cries in front of her doctor, she is practically guaranteed to be given a prescription for an antidepressant.

Psychotropic medications can be incredibly useful. They are sometimes so effective that some psychiatrists—such as Peter Kramer in his well-known book *Listening to Prozac*—have described patients whose entire personality was transformed.[8] Like all practitioners of my generation, I myself frequently prescribe psychotropic medications, especially for severe psychiatric problems. I believe that the discovery of successful psychotropic drugs is one of the major events in 20th-century medicine. But, the benefits of psychiatric medications often stop after treatment is discontinued, and a large number of patients relapse.[9] For example, a thorough Harvard study from a group that specialized in drug treatments shows that roughly half of patients who stopped taking an antidepressant relapse within a year.[10] Clearly, anti-anxiety and antidepressant medications do not "cure" in the sense that antibiotics cure infections. As such, medications, even the most useful ones, are far from an ideal solution for emotional health. In their heart of hearts, patients know this, and they often balk at taking a medication for the common problems of life, whether it is a difficult mourning or simply too much stress at work.

A Different Approach

Today, new emotional treatments are being propagated all over the world, treatments without conventional talk therapy or Prozac. For 5 years at the University of Pittsburgh's Shadyside Hospital, we have been exploring how to relieve depression, anxiety, and stress with an ensemble of natural methods that rely mainly on the natural healing mechanisms of the body rather than on language or drugs.

The main assumptions behind the work we have done can be summarized as follows:

• Inside the brain is an emotional brain, a true "brain within the brain." This second brain is built differently, it has a different cellular organization, and it even has biochemical properties that are different from the rest of the neocortex, the most "evolved" part

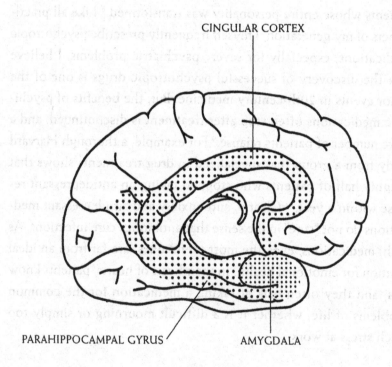

CINGULAR CORTEX

PARAHIPPOCAMPAL GYRUS   AMYGDALA

THE LIMBIC BRAIN

At the heart of the human brain is an emotional brain. These so-called "limbic" structures are the same in all mammals and are made of a different neural tissue than that of the cortical "cognitive" brain, which is responsible for language and abstract thinking. Limbic structures are responsible for emotions and the instinctual control of behavior. Deep inside the brain is the amygdala—a group of neurons responsible for the reaction of fear.

of the brain and the center of language and thought. To some degree, the emotional brain functions independently of this more
"advanced" brain. In fact, language and cognition have limited
access to the emotional brain.
- The emotional brain controls everything that governs one's psychological well-being, as well as what governs a large part of the
body's physiology: the working order of the heart, blood pressure,
hormones, the digestive system, and even the immune system.
- Emotional disorders result from dysfunctions in the emotional
brain. For many people, these dysfunctions originated with
painful past experiences that have no relation to the present yet
still continue to control their behavior.
- The primary task of treatment is to "reprogram" the emotional
brain so that it adapts to the present instead of continuing to
react to past experiences. To achieve this goal, it is generally
more effective to use methods that act via the *body* and directly
influence the emotional brain rather than use approaches that depend entirely on language and reason, to which the emotional
brain is not as receptive.
- The emotional brain contains natural mechanisms for self-healing:
an "instinct to heal." This instinct to heal encompasses the emotional brain's innate abilities to find balance and well-being, comparable to other mechanisms of self-healing in the body, like the
scarring of a wound or the elimination of an infection. Methods
that act via the body tap into these mechanisms.

The natural methods of treatment I will present in the following
pages directly impact the emotional brain, almost entirely short-
circuiting language. Although many such methods are being proposed today, in my clinical practice, and in this book, I have selected
only those that have received enough scientific attention to make me
comfortable in using them with patients and in recommending them
to my colleagues. Each of the following chapters presents one of

these approaches, illustrated by the stories of patients whose lives
have been transformed by their experience. I also try to show the degree to which each method has been scientifically evaluated. Some
of the very recent methods include "eye movement desensitization
and reprocessing" (better known as EMDR), or heart rate coherence
training, or even the synchronization of chronobiological rhythms
with artificial dawn (which should replace your alarm clock). Other
approaches, like acupuncture, nutrition, exercise, emotional communication, and cultivating your connection to something larger than
yourself, stem from age-old traditions, though new scientific data are
giving them a renewed importance.

Whatever their origins may be, everything begins with emotions.
We will start by reviewing how the emotional brain works, and how
it depends on the body for its healing.

2

Discontent in Neurobiology:
The Difficult Marriage of Two Brains

We must take care not to make intellect our god. It has, of course,
powerful muscles, but no personality. It cannot rule, only serve.

—ALBERT EINSTEIN

Without emotions, life would have no meaning. Without love, beauty, justice, truth, dignity, honor, and the satisfaction each of these provide, what would make life worth living?

These experiences, and the emotions that go with them, are like compasses. Step by step, they point us in the right direction. We are continually gravitating toward more love, more beauty, more justice, and seeking to distance ourselves from their opposites. Without emotions, we lose our fundamental bearings—we cannot make choices that reflect what truly matters most to us.

Some people with serious mental illness lose that ability. They enter a kind of emotional "no man's land." Like Peter, for example, a young Canadian who turned up in the emergency room of my hospital when I was still an intern.

For some time, Peter had been hearing voices. They had told him that he was ridiculous and incapable and would be better off dead. Little by little, the voices had taken over, and Peter's behavior had become increasingly odd. He had stopped washing, refused to eat, and remained shut up in his room for several days in a row. His mother, who lived alone with him, was terribly worried. Her only son, the brilliant philosophy student at the top of his freshman class, had always been a little eccentric. Still, this time, it all seemed excessive.

One day, in a state of exasperation, Peter had insulted and struck his mother. She had had to call the police. And that was how he arrived in the emergency room. With medication, Peter calmed down a great deal. The voices virtually disappeared within a few days. He said that he could now "control them." But that did not mean that he became normal.

After several weeks of treatment—antipsychotic medications must be taken over a long period—his mother was almost as worried as she had been on the first day. "He doesn't feel anything anymore," she told me with pleading in her voice. "Look at him. He's no longer interested in anything. He doesn't do anything anymore. He spends his days smoking and doing nothing."

I observed Peter while she spoke. He was pitiful to watch. Slightly stooped, with his frozen features and stony gaze, he walked up and down the hospital corridor like a zombie. The brilliant student had almost stopped reacting to others or to news from the outside world. This state of emotional apathy is what most inspires concern in the families of patients like Peter. Yet his hallucinations and delusions—which the medication had dispelled—were a lot more dangerous for him and his mother than these side effects. But there's the rub: no emotion, no life.*

---

*Today there are antipsychotic medications whose side effects are less disturbing. They can control hallucinations and delusions without deadening the patient's emotional life to the same degree.

On the other hand, abandoned to themselves, emotions do not make life perfect. They must be tempered by the rational analysis that the cognitive brain provides. Otherwise, rash decisions made in the heat of action can imperil the complex equilibrium of our relations with others. Deprived of concentration, thoughtfulness, planning, we are tossed about by the pleasures and frustrations that come our way by chance. If we are incapable of controlling our existence, life loses its meaning, too.

Emotional Intelligence

"Emotional intelligence" is the term that best defines this balance between emotion and reason. The term was invented by researchers from Yale and the University of New Hampshire.[1] Emotional intelligence, an idea as simple as it is important, gained its fame from a book by Daniel Goleman, a science reporter for the *New York Times*.[2] The worldwide impact of Daniel Goleman's book reawakened debate on the old question, "What is intelligence?"

The original and most general definition of intelligence was the one that inspired psychologists at the beginning of the 20th century to invent the concept of the "intelligence quotient." Intelligence, according to this view, is a set of mental capacities by which we can predict an individual's success. Generally speaking, therefore, the more "intelligent" individuals are—that is to say, the higher their IQ (intelligence quotient)—the better they should "succeed." To verify that prediction, early psychological researchers created a measure destined to become famous: the IQ test. The test evaluates, above all, an individual's capacities for abstraction and flexibility in the treatment of logical information. However, the relationship between a person's IQ and his or her "success" in a fairly broad sense (social position, income, marital status, ability to raise successful children) has turned out to be tenuous, to say the least. According to various studies, less than 20 percent of that success may be attributed to an individual's IQ.

The conclusion seems compelling: Other factors make up the remaining 80 percent of success. Therefore, these other factors are clearly more important than abstract intelligence and logic in determining success.

Carl Jung and Jean Piaget—Swiss pioneers in psychiatry and child psychology, respectively—had already suggested in the 1950s that there are several types of intelligence. Undeniably certain individuals—such as Mozart—have a remarkable "intelligence for music." Others have an unusual "intelligence for shape"—Rodin, for example—and still others for movement in space. The athlete Michael Jordan or the dancer Rudolf Nureyev come to mind.

The Yale and New Hampshire researchers revealed another form of intelligence, one involved in understanding and regulating emotions. This form of intelligence—"emotional intelligence"—is precisely the one that, more than any other, explains success in life. And it has very little to do with IQ.

The researchers at Yale and the University of New Hampshire set out to define an "emotional quotient" or "EQ" that would serve to measure this concept of emotional intelligence. They based their definition on four essential skills:

1. The capacity to identify our emotional state and that of others;
2. The ability to grasp the natural course of emotions (just as the movements of a bishop and a knight follow different rules on a chessboard, fear and anger, for example, unfold differently and have different consequences on our behavior);
3. The ability to reason about our own emotions and those of others;
4. The ability to regulate our emotions and those of others.[3]

These four aptitudes provide the basis for self-mastery and for so-cial success. Together, they form the foundation of self-knowledge, self-restraint, compassion, cooperation, and the capacity to resolve conflict. While these skills may sound elementary, and most of us are probably convinced that we have these skills, it is certainly not the case.

I remember, for example, a brilliant young researcher at the med-ical school in Pittsburgh. She had agreed to participate in an experi-ment in my laboratory on localizing emotions in the brain. In this study, the participants watched extracts of films with powerful, often violent, images, while their brains were monitored by an MRI (mag-netic resonance imaging) scanner.*

The experiment is still vivid in my mind because I had acquired a strong aversion to these films from seeing them so much. As soon as the experiment got under way, with the young woman stretched out inside the scanner, her heart rate and blood pressure rose rapidly to an abnormal degree. I was worried enough by this obvious sign of stress to offer to cancel the experiment. With an air of surprise, she answered me that everything was fine. She was not feeling anything; the images had no effect on her, she said, and she did not understand why I was offering to stop everything!

Later, I discovered that the young woman had very few friends and lived only for her work. Without really understanding why, the mem-bers of my team did not really like her. Was it because she talked too much about herself and did not seem to care about the people around her? She herself had no idea at all why she was not appreciated more.

To me, this researcher remains a typical example of a person with a high IQ and a very poor EQ. Her chief shortcoming seemed to be a lack of awareness of her own emotions and, as a result, her "blind-ness" to the emotions of others. Her career prospects looked dim to

---

*Nuclear magnetic resonance imaging can detect changes in the activity of neurons in different regions of the brain as they are impacted by the content of thoughts and emotions.

me. Even in the "hard" sciences, people have to work in teams, form bonds, exercise leadership, and cooperate with colleagues. Whatever our vocation, circumstances always call on us to interact with others. This reality is inescapable, and our capacity for relating to others determines our success in the long term.

The behavior of young children illustrates how hard it can be sometimes to identify emotional states. Crying infants usually do not know exactly why they are crying. It may be because they are hungry, too warm, sad, or simply tired after a long day of play. They cry without knowing what is wrong; they don't know what to do to feel better. In situations like these, parents with underdeveloped emotional intelligence will easily feel overwhelmed; they will not know how to identify the infant's emotion and thus respond to its need. Others with greater emotional intelligence will easily find out how to calm the child. Descriptions abound of the way T. Berry Brazelton, the outstanding pediatrician of his generation, managed, with a single word or gesture, to calm a child who had been crying for days. He is a virtuoso of emotional intelligence.

In children, this inability to distinguish clearly between different emotional states is common. But I often also observed this with residents in my hospital. Under stress after interminable workdays, and exhausted by night call several times a week, they frequently compensated by overeating. Their bodies were telling them: "I need to take a break; I need to sleep." But they only heard, "I need, I need . . ." They reacted to this demand with the only physical gratification instantly available in any hospital—the fast food at their disposal 24 hours a day. In a situation like this, using emotional intelligence would mean calling forth the four aptitudes described by the Yale study:

- First, identifying the original state for what it really is (fatigue, not hunger)

- Second, knowing how it develops (a passing state, it occurs off and on throughout the day when the body is overtaxed)
- Next, reasoning about the problem (eating one more ice cream would be an extra burden on my body; besides, it would make me feel guilty)
- Finally, taking charge of the situation in an appropriate fashion (learning to let the wave of fatigue pass over, or taking a break for "meditation" or even a 20-minute nap; we can always find time for these alternatives, which are a lot more reinvigorating than yet another cup of coffee or chocolate bar)

The case of the tired residents may seem trivial. But the situation is interesting for that exact reason. Overeating is both very ordinary and yet very hard to bring under control. Most specialists of nutrition and obesity agree on this issue: Poor mastery of emotions is one of the major causes of obesity in a society where stress is common and food is used abundantly to deal with it. People who have learned to handle stress generally do not have a weight problem. They have learned how to listen to their bodies, identify their feelings, and respond intelligently.

According to Goleman's thesis, mastering emotional intelligence is a better indicator of success in life than IQ. In one of the most remarkable studies of the factors predicting success, psychologists tracked nearly 100 Harvard students, beginning in the 1940s.[4] Their intellectual performance at 20 was a poor predictor of their future income, productivity, or recognition by their peers. Nor did those with the highest grades at university have the happiest family life or the most friends later on. In contrast, a study of children from a poor suburb of Boston suggests that "emotional quotient" plays a significant role. The most powerful predictor of these children's success as adults was not their IQ—it was their ability, during their difficult childhoods, to govern their emotions, deal with their frustration, and cooperate with others.[5]

The Third Revolution: Beyond Darwin and Freud

Two great thinkers, Darwin and Freud, dominated social sciences in the 20th century. It took nearly 100 years for their two contributions to be joined into an entirely new perspective on the emotional life of human beings.

According to Darwin, species evolve through the successive addition of new structures and functions. Every organism therefore has the physical characteristics of its ancestors, as well as new ones. Since humans and apes branched off from their common ancestors late in the course of evolution, humans are, in a sense, *"super-apes."** As for our ape ancestors, they themselves have a number of the same traits as all the other mammals with which they share a common ancestor. And so it goes, all the way up the evolutionary chain.

Like archeological excavations, the anatomy and physiology of the human brain reveal the successive layers deposited by our evolutionary past. The deep structures of the brain are identical to those of apes. Some of the deepest are even the same as those of reptiles. On the other hand, structures added more recently by evolution, such as the prefrontal cortex (behind the forehead), are only highly developed in humans. That's why the rounded forehead of *Homo sapiens* distinguishes us so clearly from the faces of our ancestors who were closer to apes. What Darwin proposed was so revolutionary and disturbing that its implications were only fully accepted toward the mid-20th century: Inside the human brain exists the brains of animals that came before us in the evolutionary chain.

Freud, for his part, defined the existence of a mysterious part of the life of the mind. He called it the "Unconscious"—what escapes not only our conscious attention but, moreover, our reasoning. Trained as a neurologist, Freud could never bring himself to admit that his theories could not be explained by the structures and func-

---

*Naturally, certain characteristics have become less pronounced, such as hairiness and protruding jaws.

tions of the brain. But, lacking the knowledge we now have of the brain's anatomy (its architecture) and, above all, of its physiology (the way it operates), he could go no further in that direction. His attempt to unify these two fields—his famous "Project for a Scientific Psychology"—ended up a failure. He was so dissatisfied with it that he refused to publish it during his lifetime. But that did not stop him from thinking constantly about it.

I remember meeting Joseph Wortis, M.D., a renowned psychiatrist, when he was 85 years old. He had gone to Vienna in the early 1930s to learn about psychoanalysis and be analyzed by Freud. Dr. Wortis later founded *Biological Psychiatry*, which became a leading scientific journal. Dr. Wortis told me how Freud had surprised him in his youth by insisting, "Don't just learn psychoanalysis as it exists today. It is already outdated. Your generation will bring about the synthesis between psychology and biology. You must devote yourself to that." While the whole world was beginning to discover his theories and his "talking cure," Freud—ever the pioneer—was already searching elsewhere.

Only at the end of the 20th century did Antonio Damasio, M.D., Ph.D.—the great American neurologist and neuroscientist who is chairman of the Department of Neurology at the University of Iowa—provide an explanation for the constant tension between the emotional and the rational brains—between passions and reason—in terms that would probably have satisfied Freud. Dr. Damasio has gone still further and also shown how emotions are quite simply indispensable to reason.

Two Brains: Cognitive and Emotional

According to Dr. Damasio, our mental life springs from a constant striving toward balance between two brains. On one hand, there is the cognitive brain—conscious, rational, and geared toward the outside world. On the other, there is the emotional brain—unconscious, primarily concerned with survival, and above all tied to the body.

Though both "brains" are obviously highly interconnected and depend on each other constantly for integrated function, they each contribute to our experience of life and to our behavior in a very different way.

As Darwin had anticipated, the human brain comprises two major parts. Deep in the brain, at its very center, lies the old, primitive brain, the one we share with all other mammals and, for the deepest nuclei, with reptiles. This brain was the first laid down by evolution. Paul Broca, the renowned 19th-century French neurologist who first described it, called it the "limbic" brain.[6] Around this limbic brain, in the course of millions of years of evolution, a much more recent layer has formed. This is the new brain, or "neocortex," meaning "new bark" or "new envelope."

THE LIMBIC BRAIN CONTROLS EMOTIONS AND THE BODY'S PHYSIOLOGY

The limbic brain is made up of the deepest layers of the human brain. In fact, to some extent it is "a brain inside the brain." An experiment done in the laboratory for clinical cognitive neuroscience at the University of Pittsburgh that I directed with Jonathan Cohen, M.D., Ph.D. (now at Princeton University), vividly illustrated this idea. When volunteers received an injection of a substance that directly stimulated the area of the brain responsible for fear (a region referred to as the "amygdala"), we saw the emotional brain become activated. The effect was similar to a lightbulb going on. Meanwhile, the neocortex surrounding the limbic brain showed no activity at all.*

During that experiment, I was the first participant injected with the substance that directly activated the emotional brain. I distinctly remember the strange feeling it provoked. I became terrified without knowing why. The experience was one of "pure" fear—fear that was related to no object in particular. Afterwards, a number of other

---

*The image of limbic structure activation is available on the Web site www.instincttoheal.org.

participants described the same strange sensation of fear, at the same time intense and "floating." Fortunately, it lasted only a few minutes.[7]

The emotional brain has a much simpler organization than the neocortex. Unlike the neocortex, most areas of the limbic brain are not organized in regular layers of neurons that would enable it to process information. To the contrary, in some of its core areas—such as the amygdala nuclei—the neurons appear to be thrown together haphazardly. Because of this more rudimentary structure, the emotional brain processes information in a much more primitive way than the cognitive brain, but it is faster and more nimble at ensuring our survival. That is why, for example, on a dark forest floor, a piece of wood resembling a snake might set off a reaction of fear. Even before the rest of the brain can determine that the object is harmless, the survival mechanism of the emotional brain will spark the response it judges best, often based on partial, incomplete, and sometimes erroneous information.[8] Even the cell tissue of the emotional brain is different from that of the neocortex.[9] When the virus of herpes or rabies attacks the brain, it infects only the limbic brain, not the neocortex. That is the reason why the first sign of rabies is highly abnormal emotional behavior.

The limbic brain is a command post that continually receives information from different parts of the body. It responds by regulating the body's physiological balance. Breathing, heart rate, blood pressure, appetite, sleep, sexual drive, the secretion of hormones, and even the immune system follow its orders. The role of the limbic brain seems to be to maintain these different functions in equilibrium. "Homeostasis" is the name that the father of modern physiology, the late-19th-century scientist Claude Bernard, gave to this state of harmony among all our physiological functions. It is the dynamic balance that keeps us alive.

From this standpoint, as the 17th-century philosopher Spinoza had intuited, and Dr. Damasio described so clearly, our emotions may be nothing more than the conscious experience of a broad set of physiological reactions overseeing *and continually adjusting* the activity of the body's biological systems to the requirements of our inner and outer environment.[10] The emotional brain is therefore almost on more intimate terms with the body than it is with the cognitive brain, which is why it is often easier to access emotions through the body than through language.

Mary Anne, for example, had been following a traditional Freudian psychoanalytic therapy for 2 years. She had lain on the couch and done her best to "free-associate" about the themes of her suffering, in particular her emotional dependence on men. She felt truly alive only when a man told her, all the time, that he loved her. She found separations, even the briefest, hard to bear; she would immediately feel a diffuse and childlike anxiety. After 2 years of analysis, Mary Anne understood her problem very well. She could describe in detail her complicated relationship with her mother, who had entrusted her to an endless stream of nursemaids. She assumed that the explanation for her deep-seated feelings of insecurity lay there. With her well-trained academic mind, she became passionately attached to analyzing her symptoms and describing them to her analyst, on whom she had naturally become . . . very dependent.

In the meantime, Mary Anne had made significant progress. She felt freer after 2 years in analysis. However, she was also aware that she had never resolved the pain and sadness of her childhood. While she had been perpetually focused on her thoughts and the words to express it, she now realized that she had never cried on the couch. She was that much more surprised, during a week at a spa, when a massage suddenly brought back the emotions of childhood.

She was lying on her back while the massage therapist gently massaged her abdomen. When the therapist approached a particular spot below her navel, Mary Anne felt a lump in her throat. The massage therapist noticed it and asked Mary Anne to merely observe what she was feeling. Then the therapist calmly persisted with circular movements precisely on that spot. A few seconds later, Mary Anne was shaken by violent sobs. She saw herself, at age 7, in the recovery room of a hospital, all alone after she had been operated on for appendicitis. Her mother had not come back from vacation to take care of her. This emotion, which she had long tried to locate in her head, had been there all along, hidden in her body.

Because of the emotional brain's close relationship with the body, it is often easier to act on it through the body rather than through language. Medications, of course, interfere directly with the functioning of neurons. But we can also mobilize intrinsic physiological rhythms such as eye movements associated with dreams, the natural variations of the heart rate, the sleep cycle, and its reliance on the rhythms of day and night. We can use physical exercise or acupuncture. Or we can master nutrition. As we shall see, emotional relationships—even our connection to others in our community—have a major physical component, a direct impact on our physical being. These physical gateways into the emotional brain are more direct and often more powerful than thought and language.

THE CORTICAL BRAIN CONTROLS COGNITION, LANGUAGE, AND REASONING

The neocortex, the "new bark," is the folded surface that gives the brain its characteristic appearance. It is also the envelope surrounding the emotional brain. The neocortex is on the brain's surface because, from an evolutionary standpoint, it is the most recent layer. The neocortex comprises six distinct strata of neurons that are perfectly regular and, like a microprocessor, organized for optimal information processing.

Even with all the recent advances in technology, today we still find it hard to program computers to recognize human faces viewed from different angles and in different lighting. But the neocortex manages to do it easily within a few milliseconds. The neocortex also has extraordinary means of processing sound. For example, the brain of a human fetus distinguishes between its maternal language and all other languages, even before birth.[11]

In humans, the area of neocortex located behind the forehead, right above the eyes, is called the "prefrontal cortex." This section is particularly well-developed. The size of the emotional brain usually varies little from one species to another (proportionate to the overall body size of each species, of course); the prefrontal cortex, however, represents a much larger proportion of the brain in humans than in all other animals.

The prefrontal cortex is the part of the neocortex responsible for attention, concentration, the inhibition of impulses and instincts, the regulation of social relations, and—as Dr. Damasio has shown— moral behavior. Above all, the neocortex makes plans for the future based on "symbols" that are only in the mind and are not visible to the eyes nor able to be felt with our hands. By controlling attention, concentration, elaboration of future plans, moral behavior, and language, the neocortex—our cognitive brain—is an essential component of our humanity.

When the Two Brains Don't Get Along

The two brains—the emotional and cognitive—take in information from the outside world more or less simultaneously. From that moment on, they can either cooperate or compete over the control of thinking, emotions, and behavior. The result of that interaction—cooperation or competition—determines what we feel, our relations with the world, and our relationships with others. Competition between the two, whatever form it takes, makes us unhappy.

When the emotional and the cognitive brains work together, however, we feel just the opposite—an inner harmony. The emotional brain directs us toward the experiences we seek, and the cognitive brain tries to get us there as intelligently as possible. From the resulting harmony comes the feeling, "I am where I want to be in my life." This feeling underlies all lasting experiences of well-being.

THE EMOTIONAL SHORT-CIRCUIT

Evolution has its own priorities. And evolution is, above all, a matter of survival and transmission of our genes from one generation to the next. While it was all very well for the brain to have developed prodigious capacities for concentration, abstraction, and reflection over the past several million years, if these capacities had prevented us from detecting the presence of a tiger or an enemy, or made us miss a chance to encounter an appropriate sexual partner and thus reproduce, our species would have long since died out.

Fortunately, the emotional brain has remained constantly on guard. Its role is to keep watch, in the background, on its surroundings. When it perceives a danger or an exceptional opportunity—a potential partner or territory, or a valuable asset—it sets off an alarm. Within a few milliseconds, the emotional brain has canceled all operations and interrupted activities in the cognitive brain. This reaction enables the whole brain to instantly concentrate its full resources on the essentials of survival. When we are driving, for example, this mechanism helps us to unconsciously detect a truck heading toward us, even while we are in the midst of a conversation with our passenger. The emotional brain identifies the danger, then focuses our attention away from the conversation and on the truck until the danger has passed. It is also the emotional brain that interrupts a conversation between two men at an outdoor café when an enticing miniskirt comes into view. It suspends conversation between two parents sitting in a playground when out of the corner of their eyes they have detected an unfamiliar dog approaching their child.

At Yale University, the laboratory of Patricia Goldman-Rakic, Ph.D., has suggested that the emotional brain can put the prefrontal cortex "off-line." Under stress, the prefrontal cortex no longer

responds and loses its capacity to control behavior. Suddenly, reflexes and instinctive responses take over.[12] These responses are
faster and closer to our genetic inheritance, and evolution has given
them priority in emergencies, where they are intentionally better
than abstract reflection at guiding us when survival is at stake.

In the early life of humans, which was closer to that of animals, this
alarm system was essential. A hundred thousand years after the emer-
gence of *Homo sapiens*, this reaction is still enormously useful in everyday
life. However, when our emotions are too strong, the predominance of
the emotional over the cognitive brain begins to take over our mental
functioning. We then lose control over the flow of our thoughts, and
we do not act in our best long-term interests. In fact, we find ourselves
being "too emotional," or even "irrational."

In medical practice, we see two common examples of emotional
short-circuiting. What we call "posttraumatic stress disorder" (PTSD)
is the first. After a serious trauma—for example, surviving a rape or an
earthquake—the emotional brain acts like a loyal and conscientious
sentry that has been caught off guard. PTSD sets off the alarm much
too often, as if the emotional brain cannot be sure that everything is
safe. We saw this happening to a survivor of September 11 who came
to our center in Pittsburgh for treatment. Months after the attack, her
body became paralyzed as soon as she entered a skyscraper.

The second common example of emotional short-circuiting is that
of anxiety attacks, which psychiatrists also call panic attacks. In indus-
trialized countries, nearly 1 person in 20 has suffered from anxiety
attacks.[13] Often the symptoms are so overwhelming that victims believe that they are about to have a heart attack. The limbic brain suddenly takes over all of the body's functions. The heart beats too fast;
the stomach tightens; legs and hands tremble; the whole body breaks
out in sweat. At the same time, a flood of adrenalin knocks out cognitive functions. The cognitive brain may very well perceive that there

is no reason for this state of alarm. But as long as it remains "off-line," it will not be able to organize a coherent response to the situation. People who have experienced such attacks describe this sensation very clearly: "My brain felt empty; I couldn't think. The only words I heard myself saying were, 'I'm dying—call an ambulance—right away!'"

COGNITIVE SMOTHERING

On the other hand, the cognitive brain controls conscious attention and does have the ability to temper emotional reactions before they get out of proportion. This regulation of the emotions by the cognitive brain frees us from the potential tyranny of emotion and a life totally controlled by instincts and reflexes. A study at Stanford University using cerebral imaging clearly reveals this role of the cortical brain. When students look at distressing photographs—of mutilated bodies or disfigured faces, for example—their emotional brain immediately reacts. However, if they make a conscious effort to control their emotions, the images of their brain in action show that the neocortical regions dominate. These areas block the activity of the emotional brain.[14]

Cognitive control, however, is a double-edged sword. If overused, it may lose contact with calls for help from the emotional brain. We often see the effects of that excessive stifling of emotion in individuals who have learned as children that their feelings were not acceptable. A commonplace example in this domain is probably the injunction men have so often heard: "Boys don't cry."

Excessive control of emotions may foster a temperament that is not "sensitive" enough. A brain that does not take information about emotions into account will face other problems. On one hand, it is much harder to make decisions when we do not feel "deep down" preferences—that is, in our heart or "gut." These are the parts of the body that give a "visceral" resonance to emotions. That is why we may sometimes see engineering types who get lost in infinitesimal detail when it comes to choosing between two cars, for example, or even two movies. Not in touch with their "gut reaction," their reasoning alone is unable to distinguish between two options that are very comparable.

In the most extreme cases, a neurological lesion prevents the cognitive brain from being aware of emotional reactions altogether. Such is the famous 19th-century example of Phineas Gage, a railroad worker whose prefrontal cortex was the only thing damaged by a tamping iron that flew through the front of his skull, miraculously leaving him alive.[15] Paul Eslinger, Ph.D., and Dr. Damasio described a modern version of Phineas Gage, with a similar type of damage to the brain.[16] "E.V.R." was an accountant endowed with an IQ of 130, placing him in the range of "superior intelligence." As a valued member of his community, he had been married for many years, had several children, attended church regularly, and led a steady life. One day he had to undergo a brain operation that resulted in "disconnecting" his cognitive brain from his emotional brain. From one day to the next, he became incapable of making even minor decisions. None of them made any "sense" to him. He could only reason about decisions in an abstract fashion. Strangely enough, IQ tests—which, in fact, measure only abstract reasoning—still showed his "intelligence" to be distinctly higher than average. Despite this, E.V.R. no longer knew how to spend his time. Deprived of genuine, visceral preferences for one or another option, all choices got confused in endless questions of detail. Finally, he lost his job. Soon thereafter, his marriage collapsed, and he got involved in a succession of questionable business deals. In the end, he lost all his money. Without emotions to guide him in his choices, his behavior was totally disordered, even though his intelligence remained intact.[17]

Even people whose brains are intact may experience serious damage to their health because they tend to stifle emotions too much. The separation between the cognitive and the emotional brains creates an extraordinary capacity to remain unaware of the small alarm bells going off in our limbic brain. For example, we can find a multitude of good reasons to cling to a marriage or a profession that, in fact, offends our deepest values and makes us unhappy day after day. But our deafness to an underlying distress does not make it go away. Since our emotional brain interacts principally with our body, this impasse may express itself in physical problems, the symptoms of which are the classic stress disorders: unexplained fatigue, high blood pressure, chronic colds and other infections, heart diseases, intestinal disorders, and skin problems. Researchers at the University of California at Berkeley have even suggested recently that the *suppression* of negative emotions by the cognitive brain, rather than the negative emotions themselves, weighs more heavily on our hearts and arteries.[18]

The State of "Flow" and the Buddha's Smile

To live in harmony in human society, we need to find and sustain a balance. This equilibrium is between our immediate—instinctive—emotional reactions and the rational responses that preserve our social ties over the long term. Emotional intelligence is best expressed when the two systems—the cortical and the limbic brain—constantly cooperate. In this state, our thoughts, decisions, and movements blend and flow naturally, without particular attention paid to them. At every moment we know what choice we should make. We pursue our objectives effortlessly, with natural concentration, because our actions are in harmony with our values. This state of well-being is what we continually aspire to. It is the sign of perfect harmony between the emotional brain, supplying energy and guidance, and the cognitive brain, bringing it to fruition. The psychologist Mihaly Csikszentmihalyi (pronounced "sheek-sent-meehal") grew up in the chaos of postwar Hungary and has devoted his life to understanding the essence of well-being. He named this condition of harmony the state of "flow."[19]

As it turns out, we have a simple physiological marker for that cerebral harmony—the smile. Darwin examined its biological foundation more than a century ago. A forced smile—a smile produced for social circumstance—mobilizes only the zygomatic muscles around the mouth, uncovering the teeth. A "real" smile, on the other hand, also mobilizes the muscles around the eyes. This second set of muscles does not contract at will, on orders from the cognitive brain. The order must come from the deep, primitive, limbic regions. That explains why the eyes themselves never lie—their folds tell us whether the smile is genuine. A warm smile, a real one, lets us know intuitively that the person we are talking to is, at that exact moment, in a state of harmony with what he or she thinks and feels, between cognition and emotion. The brain has the innate ability to attain the state of flow, a universal symbol of which can be seen in the smile on Buddha's face.

The purpose of the natural methods that I am going to set forth in the following chapters is to promote that harmony or to recover it once it has been lost. In contrast to IQ, which changes very little in the course of a lifetime, our emotional intelligence can be cultivated at any age. It is never too late to learn how to govern our emotions and our relations with others. The first approach I describe here is probably the most fundamental. By learning how to optimize our own heart rhythm, we can learn to withstand stress, control anxiety, and maximize our vital energy. And this one key technique just may give us clues into the underlying links between many methods of emotional healing.

3

The Heart and Its Reasons

"Goodbye," said the fox. "Here is my secret. It's quite simple: one sees clearly only with the heart."

—ANTOINE DE SAINT-EXUPÉRY, *THE LITTLE PRINCE*,
TRANSLATED BY RICHARD HOWARD

The conductor Herbert von Karajan once said that he lived only for music. He probably did not know how true that would turn out to be: He died the same year that he retired, after 30 years directing the Berlin Philharmonic Orchestra. But what is even more surprising is that two Austrian psychologists could have predicted it. Twelve years earlier, they had examined how the maestro's heart reacted as he pursued various activities.[1] The greatest variations in von Karajan's heart rate were recorded while he was conducting a particularly emotional passage from Beethoven's *Lenora Overture No. 3*. In fact, he had only to hear this particular passage again in order to experience practically the same acceleration in his heartbeat.

In that composition, other passages are far more physically demanding. Yet they provoked only a slight increase in von Karajan's heart rate. As for his other activities, von Karajan seemed to take them less to heart, so to speak. Whether he was landing his private plane or simulating an emergency re-takeoff, his heart hardly seemed to notice. Karajan's heart was given over entirely to music. And when the maestro gave up music, his heart gave out.

Who has not heard the story of an elderly neighbor who died a few months after his wife? Or a great aunt whose death followed soon after the loss of her son? It was commonly said that they had "died of a broken heart." Medical science used to treat such descriptions with disdain, attributing these incidents to simple coincidence. Only recently, over the last 20 years, have several teams of cardiologists and psychiatrists taken a close look at such "anecdotes." They have discovered that stress is possibly an even greater risk factor for heart disease than smoking.[2] They have also found that an episode of depression coming within six months of a myocardial infarction is a more accurate predictor of death than most measurements of heart function.[3]

When the emotional brain is out of order, the heart suffers and wears out. But the most astonishing discovery of all is that this relationship works both ways. The proper functioning of the heart turns out to influence the brain as well. Some cardiologists and neurologists go so far as to refer to a "heart-brain system" that cannot be dissociated.[4]

If there were a medication capable of harmonizing this intimate interplay between the heart and brain, it would have beneficial effects on the whole body. This miracle drug might slow down aging, reduce stress and fatigue, overcome anxiety, and shield us from depression. At night, it would help us to sleep better, and in the daytime, to function more effectively, enhancing our capacities for concentration and performance. Above all, by adjusting the balance between the brain and the rest of the body, the drug would help us foster the sense of "flow" that is synonymous with well-being. This one medication could be an antihypertensive, an anxiolytic (anti-anxiety drug) and an anti-depressant all in one. If such a medication existed, not a single doctor would fail to prescribe it. Like fluoride for teeth, governments might even end up putting it in our drinking water.

Alas, this miracle drug does not yet exist. Or does it? A simple and effective method available to all of us seems to create the very conditions essential for harmony between the brain and heart. Although this method has only recently been described, several studies have already shown beneficial effects. Good for the body as well as the emotions of those who have mastered it, this method's effects even include a partial reversal of physiological aging. To understand how it works, we first need to briefly examine how the heart-brain system functions.

The Heart of Emotions

We experience emotions in our body, not in our head. Already in 1890, William James, a Harvard professor and the father of American psychology, wrote that an emotion was first of all a physical state and only accessorily a perception in the brain. He based his conclusions on the ordinary experience of emotions. Don't we speak of fear as "having your heart in your throat?" or of gaiety as feeling "light-hearted?" or of bad temper as "bile?" It would be a mistake to consider these expressions as mere figures of speech. They are fairly exact representations of what we experience when we find ourselves in different emotional states.*

---

*In his remarkable book *Looking for Spinoza: Joy, Sorrow and the Feeling Brain* (Harcourt, Inc., 2003), Antonio Damasio, M.D., Ph.D., expands greatly on this idea. He also reminds readers that Baruch Spinoza—the great 16th-century philosopher—anticipated the neurological discoveries that would come much later, at the end of the 20th century.

In fact, only recently was it discovered that the digestive system and the heart have their own network of tens of thousands of neurons that act like "small brains" in the body. Like individual regions in the brain itself (so-called "nuclei"), these local brains have their own perceptions. Though their processing capacities are limited, these groups of neurons are also capable of adapting their behavior according to these perceptions, and even of changing their responses as a result of their experience—that is, in a certain sense, of creating their own memories.[5]

Besides possessing its own network of semiautonomous neurons, the heart is also a small hormone factory. It produces its own supply of adrenalin, which it releases when it needs to function at maximum capacity. The heart makes and controls the release of another hormone, ANF (atrial natriuretic factor), which regulates blood pressure. It secretes its own reserves of oxytocin, often called the love peptide. (This hormone is released into the blood, for example, when a mother breastfeeds her child, during courtship, and with orgasms.[6]) All these hormones act directly on the brain. Finally, the heart may affect the whole organism through the variations of its electromagnetic field, which can be detected several feet away from the body, but whose significance we do not yet understand.[7]

Clearly, the references to the heart in the words we use to describe our emotions are more than mere metaphors. The heart perceives and feels. It partly sets its own course of action. And when it expresses itself, it influences the physiology of our whole body, including the brain.

To Marie, these considerations were far from theoretical. At 50, she had been suffering for several years from sudden anxiety attacks, which could catch her by surprise anywhere and anytime. First, her heart would start to beat too fast, much too fast. One day at a party, her heart started to race. To keep from falling, she had to hang on to the arm of a man she didn't even know. This constant uncertainty about the way her heart would react made her very uncomfortable.

She began to restrict her activities. After the cocktail party incident, she stopped going out unless she was accompanied by her daughter or close friends. She no longer drove alone to her country house for fear of her heart, in her words, "giving out."

Marie had no idea what set off these attacks. It was as if her heart decided all of a sudden that it was terrified of something she was not aware of. Her thoughts then became confused and anxious and she started to feel shaky on her legs.

Her cardiologist diagnosed a "mitral valve prolapse," a mild affliction, which, she was told, should give her nothing to worry about. He prescribed beta-blocker medication to prevent her heart from racing, but this led to fatigue and gave her nightmares. She made the decision to stop taking her medicine, without telling her doctor.

When she came to see me, I had just read an article in the *American Journal of Psychiatry* showing how patients with such symptoms often responded well to treatment with antidepressants,[8] as if the uncontrolled acceleration originated in the brain rather than with the abnormal valve. Unfortunately, my treatment was scarcely more effective than my cardiologist colleague's. Besides, Marie was very unhappy about the extra pounds she put on because of her new medication. Marie's heart calmed down only when she learned to tame it directly. I would almost say, "when she learned to listen and speak to it."

The relationship between the emotional brain and the "small brain" in the heart is one of the keys to emotional mastery. By learning—literally—how to control our heart, we learn how to gain mastery of our emotional brain, and vice versa. The strongest relationship between the heart and the emotional brain is a diffuse two-way communication network known as the "autonomic peripheral nervous system." This is part of the nervous system that—beyond our conscious control—regulates the functioning of our organs.

The autonomic nervous system is made up of two branches, beginning at the emotional brain and spreading throughout the body. The "sympathetic" branch releases adrenalin and noradrenalin, regulating reactions of "fight or flight." The autonomic nervous system's activity speeds up the heart rate.* The other branch, called "parasympathetic," releases a different neurotransmitter—acetylcholine—that promotes states of relaxation and calm, and slows down the heart.[†]

In mammals, these two systems—the accelerator and the brake— are constantly in balance. That balance is what enables mammals to adapt very rapidly to the vast potential for changes that may occur in their environment. When a rabbit is safely chewing on the grass in front of its hole, it can stop at any moment, raise its head, prick up its ears, scan the horizon like radar, and sniff the air to detect a predator's presence. Once the danger signal has vanished, it quickly goes back to its meal.

Only mammals have such a flexible physiology. To negotiate the unforeseen twists and turns of existence, we need both a brake and an accelerator. They need to be in perfect working order, and they have to be equally strong to counterbalance each other, if the need arises (see "The Heart-Brain System," page 39).

According to researcher Stephen Porges, Ph.D., of the University of Maryland, the delicate balance between the two branches of the autonomic nervous system has enabled mammals to develop increasingly complex social relations in the course of evolution. The most complex among them seems to be love relationships, especially the particularly delicate phase of courtship. When a man or woman in whom we are interested looks at us and our heart beats wildly or we start to blush, it is because our sympathetic system has stepped on the accelerator, perhaps a little too much. If we take a deep breath to recover our poise and carry on the conversation, we have just pressed on

---

*The term "sympathetic" comes from the Latin root meaning "to be in relation" because the nerve branches run along the side of the spinal cord, which is encased in the spinal column.

[†]The neurotransmitter of the parasympathetic system is acetylcholine.

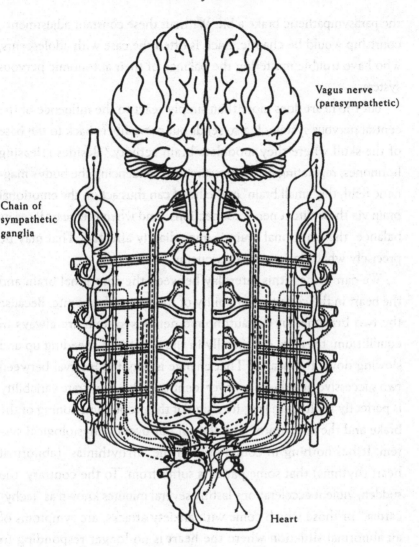

Vagus nerve
(parasympathetic)

Chain of
sympathetic
ganglia

Heart

THE HEART-BRAIN SYSTEM

*The semi-independent network of neurons that constitutes the "small brain in the heart" is
closely connected with the brain itself. Together, they make up a true "heart-brain system."
Within this system, the two organs constantly influence each other. Among the mechanisms
connecting the heart and the brain, the autonomic nervous system plays a particularly important role. It has two branches: the "sympathetic" branch speeds up the heart and activates the
emotional brain; the "parasympathetic" branch acts as a brake on both.*

the parasympathetic brake a bit. Without these constant adjustments, courtship would be chaotic. Such is often the case with adolescents, who have trouble mastering the balance of their autonomic nervous system.

But the heart does more than simply react to the influence of the central nervous system: It also sends out nerve fibers back to the base of the skull where they modulate brain activity.[9] Besides releasing hormones, regulating blood pressure, and influencing the body's magnetic field, the "small brain" in the heart can thus act on the emotional brain via these direct nerve connections. And when the heart loses its balance, the emotional brain is immediately affected. That may be precisely what Marie was experiencing.

We can witness this interplay between the emotional brain and the heart in the constant variability of the normal heart rate. Because the two branches of the autonomic nervous system are always in equilibrium, they are continually in the process of speeding up and slowing down the heart.[10] That change is why the interval between two successive heartbeats is never identical. This heart rate variability is perfectly healthy; in fact, it's a sign of the proper functioning of the brake and the accelerator, and thus of our overall physiological system. It has nothing in common with the "arrhythmias" (abnormal heart rhythms) that some patients suffer from. To the contrary, the sudden, violent accelerations lasting several minutes known as "tachycardia," or those which come with anxiety attacks, are symptoms of an abnormal situation where the heart is no longer responding to modulation from the parasympathetic brake.

On the opposite extreme, when the heart beats like a metronome without the slightest variability, the situation is particularly serious. Obstetricians were the first to recognize it: During childbirth, they learned to keep a very close eye on any fetus with an excessively regular heart rate because it suggests a potentially fatal problem. We now know that this is true of adults as well. The heart begins to beat with such great regularity only when we approach death.

Chaos and Coherence

I discovered my own "heart-brain system" on the display of a laptop computer. The tip of my finger was slipped into a ring connected to the machine. The computer simply measured the interval between each heartbeat detected on the pad of my index finger. When the interval was a little shorter—my heart having beaten a little faster—a blue line on the screen went up a notch. When the interval was longer—my heart having slowed down a little—the line turned back down.

On the screen, I saw the blue line zigzagging up and down for no apparent reason. With each heartbeat, my heart seemed to be making adjustments. But there was no structure in the peaks and dips as my heart accelerated and slowed down. The curve looked like a series of crests in a distant mountain range. Even if my heart was beating an average of 62 beats a minute, it could climb to 70 and drop back down to 55 from one moment to the next, for no discernable reason.

The technician reassured me. This zigzag was, she said, the normal pattern of heart rate variability. She then asked me to start counting aloud: "Subtract 9 from 1,356, then continue subtracting 9 from each new figure you get. . . ." While this task was not too hard to do, being put to the test in front of a small group of observers who were there, like me, to satisfy their curiosity about the machine was not particularly pleasant. Immediately, to my great surprise, the curve became even more jagged and the average number of heartbeats jumped to 72. Ten beats more a minute, simply because I was handling a few figures! What an energy guzzler, the brain! Or perhaps it was the stress of having to do arithmetic in public?

The curve had become even more irregular as my heartbeat accelerated, so the cause was likely to be anxiety rather than mere mental effort, the technician explained. Yet I did not feel anything. She then asked me to focus my attention on my heart and to bring to mind a pleasant or happy memory. I was surprised by her request.

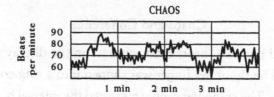

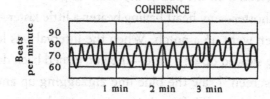

CHAOS AND COHERENCE

In states of stress, anxiety, depression, or anger, the variability between consecutive heartbeats becomes irregular, or "chaotic," and it has no internal structure. In states of well-being, compassion, or gratitude, this variability becomes "coherent"—the heart rate alternates regularly between speeding up and slowing down. Coherence maximizes the variation within a given interval of time and produces greater—and healthier—heart rate variability. (This picture is derived from the "Freeze-Framer" software produced by the HeartMath Institute in Boulder Creek, California.)

I knew that she was coaching me to calm down. But generally, reaching a state of inner calm using the techniques of meditation or relaxation requires that you empty your mind, not think about pleasant memories. But I did what she asked, and in a few seconds, the line on the screen changed radically: The sharp turns, the mountains and valleys, had changed into a series of gentle wavelets, and then stronger waves that were regular, smooth, and shapely. My heart seemed to alternate between a gentle accelerating and slowing down. Its rate ebbed and flowed with the calm rhythm of waves lapping the shore. Like an athlete who tenses and relaxes his muscles before making an effort, my heart seemed to be confidently showing that it could do both and as often as it wanted to. The window at the bottom of the screen indicated that my physiology had gone from 100 percent "chaos" to 80 percent "coherence." And all I had had to do to produce this result was to recall a pleasant memory while concentrating on my heart!

Over the past 10 years, software like the program I have just described has become capable of demonstrating two characteristic modes of variation in cardiac rhythm—chaos and coherence. Usually variations are weak and "chaotic." The heart steps on the accelerator and puts on the brake erratically; the pattern of beats is jumbled, disorderly. On the other hand, when heart rate variability is strong and healthy, the phases of accelerating and slowing down alternate rapidly and regularly. This produces the image of a harmonious wave, which is appropriately described as "coherence" of heart rate variability.

Between birth, when it is greatest, and the time of approaching death, when it is slightest, the variability of our heart rate declines about 3 percent a year.[11] Our physiology loses its flexibility little by little and finds it harder and harder to adapt to the variations in our physical and emotional surroundings. This loss of variability is a sign of aging. When variability declines, it is partly because we are not maintaining our physiological brake, the healthy "tone" of our parasympathetic system. Like an unused muscle, this system atrophies progressively over the years. Meanwhile, we never stop using our accelerator—the sympathetic system. Thus, after decades of this mode of operation, our physiology has become like a car that can suddenly pick up speed or coast downhill in neutral but has become virtually incapable of adjusting to road turns. The decline in heart rate variability correlates with an entire set of health problems related to stress and aging: high blood pressure, heart failure, complications from diabetes, myocardial infarctions, arrhythmias, sudden death, and even cancer. And studies published in such prestigious and authoritative journals as *The Lancet* and *Circulation* (the journal published by the American Heart Association) confirm this. In *Circulation*, James Nolan, M.D., and his colleagues concluded a study of 433 patients with moderate heart failure with the following statement: "A reduction in SDNN (heart rate variability) identifies patients at high risk of death and is a better predictor of death due to progressive heart failure than other conventional clinical measurements."

When variability has ceased, when the heart no longer responds to our emotions and, above all, when it can no longer "slow down" appropriately, death is near.[12]

A Day in Charles's Life

At 40, Charles is the manager of an important department store. He has climbed the corporate ladder and he is perfectly comfortable in his field. The only problem is that for months he has suffered from "palpitations." They cause him considerable worry and have led him to see several cardiologists, who have not succeeded in helping him. He has now reached the point where he has made up his mind to stop practicing sports. He is afraid he might set off an attack that would lead him once more to the emergency room. He also keeps an eye on himself when he makes love to his wife for fear of straining his heart. In his opinion, his working conditions are "perfectly normal" and "not exceptionally stressful." He nevertheless explains, in the course of our sessions, that he's thinking of resigning from his prestigious position. The reality is that the president of the corporation is often contemptuous and cynical. Although Charles has functioned well in this competitive—often aggressive—setting, he has remained a sensitive person who is wounded by the harsh, disagreeable comments of his president. Moreover, as often happens, the president's cynicism rubs off on all the other members of the team: Charles's colleagues in marketing, advertising, and finance maintain chilly relations with each other and are often abrasive in their remarks.

Charles agreed to record the variability of his heart rate over a 24-hour period. In order to analyze the results, he had to write down his different activities throughout the day. Interpreting the outcome was not very difficult. At 11 in the morning, calm, concentrated, and efficient, he was choosing photographs for a catalogue, seated at his desk. His heart rhythm demonstrated healthy coherence. Then, at noon, his heart rhythm shifted into a chaos mode, in addition to speeding up by about 12 beats a minute. At that moment, he was heading toward his president's office. One minute later, his heart was beating even faster and the chaos was total. That state was to prevail for two hours: He had just been told that the development strategy he had taken a number of weeks to prepare was "worthless." If he was not capable of organizing it more clearly, perhaps he should hand the project over to someone else to take care of. After leaving the president's office, Charles had a typical episode of palpitations that forced him to leave the building to calm down.

In the afternoon, Charles had a meeting. The recording showed another episode of chaos lasting more than 30 minutes. When I questioned him, Charles was first incapable of remembering what could have brought it on. Upon reflection, though, he recalled that the marketing director had commented, without looking at him, that the look and feel of the catalogs currently being produced didn't fit the new image the store was trying to promote. But when he was back in his office, the chaos abated and gave way to a relative coherence. At that moment, Charles was busy reviewing a production plan he had great faith in. In a traffic jam on his way home that evening, his irritation brought on another episode of chaos. Once he arrived home, he embraced his wife and children, and that was followed by a 10-minute phase of coherence. Why only 10 minutes? Because after that, Charles turned on the television to watch the news.

Different research has shown that negative emotions, such as anger, anxiety, sadness, and even ordinary worries, reduce cardiac variability the most and sow chaos in our physiology.[13] In contrast, positive emotions, like joy, gratitude, and, especially, love, appear to promote the greatest coherence. Within a few seconds, these emotions induce a wave of coherence immediately visible in the recording of cardiac frequency.[14] For Charles, as for the rest of us, the chaotic passages in our daily physiology produce a real loss of vital energy. In a study involving several thousand executives from large European corporations, more than 70 percent of them described themselves as "tired," either "most of the time" or "all the time." And 50 percent of them frankly said they were "exhausted."[15] How can competent and enthusiastic men and women, whose work is an essential part of their identity, get to this point? It may be precisely the accumulation of chaotic passages they hardly notice. These daily aggressions to their emotional balance, when sustained over the long term, drain their energy, which may lead to dreaming of a different job or, in our personal realm, of another family, another life.

Happily, in contrast with our experiences with chaos, we all experience passages of coherence as well. They do not necessarily stand out as crowning moments of existence, such as instants of ecstasy or rapture, that leave a mark. In a laboratory in California where cardiac coherence is researched, Josh, the 12-year-old son of one of the engineers, often stopped in to see his father and his team. He always brought along Mabel, his Labrador. One day, the engineers had the idea of measuring Josh and Mabel's cardiac coherence. Away from each other, Josh and Mabel were in a perfectly ordinary half-chaotic, half-coherent state. As soon as they were together, they were both in a state of coherence. If they were then separated, the coherence vanished once again, almost immediately. For Josh and Mabel, merely being together generated coherence. They must have felt it intuitively, because they were inseparable. To them, being together was surely not an extraordinary experience, but simply one that constantly nurtured their emotional being, something that did them good. Something that meant that Josh never wondered if he should spend his life with a different dog, or Mabel with a different master. Their relationship brought them an inner coherence; it sounded a chord in their hearts.

The state of cardiac coherence influences other physiological rhythms. In particular, the natural variability in blood pressure and in respiratory rhythms rapidly synchronizes with cardiac coherence. These three systems operate in unison.

This phenomenon is comparable to the phase alignment of light waves in a laser beam, which, for that very reason, is called "coherence." This alignment provides the laser with its energy and power. A 100-watt lightbulb dissipates its energy in every direction and loses its effectiveness, but when focused into a beam and phase-aligned, this same amount of light can pierce a sheet of metal. The coherence of cardiac variability may save energy in the same manner. This focusing of energy is probably why, 6 months after a training session in cardiac coherence, 80 percent of the executives cited above no longer said they were "exhausted." Only one in six of those who earlier stated they suffered from insomnia still had trouble sleeping. Only one in eight who had described themselves as "tense" continued to do so. Reducing the useless waste of energy may really be all that is needed to restore natural vitality.

In Charles's case, a few computer-aided training sessions in coherence enabled him to control his palpitations. There's nothing magic or mysterious about his progress. Every day, he did a few exercises by himself to practice experiencing the feelings in his chest that go with coherence, and in between, he remembered to evoke these same feelings whenever he started noticing tension building up in the course of his day. By doing so, he considerably reinforced the balance of his sympathetic and parasympathetic systems. In other words, he strengthened and adjusted the timing of his physiological brake.

Like a well-trained athlete's muscles, once this brake is "in shape," it becomes increasingly easy to use. With a finely tuned brake that can be counted on to work at all times, our physiology does not skid out of control, even when outside circumstances are difficult. Two months after his first session, Charles was once again practicing sports and making love to his wife with the enthusiasm that their relationship deserved. Facing his president, he had learned to remain focused on the sensations in his chest in order to maintain his coherence and to prevent his physiology from getting carried away. In fact, he was now able to answer with more tact. He could also find the words to neutralize his colleagues' aggression without being defensive (more about this in chapter 12).

Stress Management

In laboratory experiences, coherence enables the brain to work faster and more accurately.[16] In everyday life, we experience this as a state in which our ideas flow naturally and effortlessly: We easily find the words to say what we want to say, and our movements are sure and effective. It is also a state in which we adapt easily to unforeseen circumstances, whatever they may be. Our physiology is in balance, open on the world, capable of finding solutions as the need arises. Coherence, therefore, is not a state of relaxation in the conventional sense of the word: It does not require that we cut ourselves off from the world, nor does it mean that our surroundings have to be static or even calm. On the contrary, in the state of coherence, we have a better hold on the outside world. You could almost say that while in coherence, we grapple hand-to-hand with exterior circumstances, but it is a harmonious, not hostile, engagement.

For example, a study of 5-year-old children whose parents had divorced helped researchers in Seattle demonstrate the impact of the children's physiological balance on their future development. Three years later, those whose cardiac variability was greatest before the divorce—and who thus had the greatest capacity to achieve coherence—were by far the least affected by the family breakup.[17] These children were also the ones who had preserved the greatest capacity for showing affection, for cooperation with others, as well as for concentration in their schoolwork.

Celeste explained to me how she used the coherence of her cardiac rhythm very clearly. At the age of 9, she was terrified at the idea of changing schools. A few weeks before the first day of school, she started to bite her nails, refused to play with her little sister, and even got up several times during the night. When I asked what situations made her most want to bite her nails, she replied immediately, "When I think about the new school." Still, she learned very quickly, as often happens with children, to focus her mind in order to control her heart rhythm (as the computer software confirmed). Some time later, she told me that she was fitting into the new school very well: "When I'm stressed, I just go into my heart and talk to the little fairy inside. She tells me that everything is going to be fine and sometimes she even tells me what I should say or what I ought to do." I smiled as I listened to her. Wouldn't we all like to have a little fairy always at our side?

Managing Stress with the Heart

The concept of cardiac coherence and the fact that it is possible to learn to easily control it runs completely counter to conventional wisdom regarding stress management. We know that chronic stress produces anxiety and depression. It also has a negative impact on the body: insomnia, wrinkles, high blood pressure, palpitations, backache, skin and digestive problems, chronic infections, infertility, sexual impotence, all caused or worsened by stress. Ultimately, chronic stress affects social relations and professional performance by promoting irritability, poor capacity for listening to others, weaker concentration, withdrawal, and loss of team spirit. These symptoms are typical of what is generally referred to as "burnout." While this term is frequently applied to work, it just as commonly results from feeling trapped in an emotional relationship that saps all our energy. In such situations, the most common reaction is usually to focus on external conditions. People say, "If only I could change my situation, I would feel much better about myself and my body would function better."

In the meantime, we grit our teeth. We look forward to the coming weekend or vacation. We dream of better days "afterwards." Everything will work out "after I have finally finished school . . . after I get another job . . . after the children leave home . . . after I've left my husband . . . after I retire. . . ." Unfortunately, things rarely work out like that. Similar problems are likely to resurface in our new situation. The dream of a Garden of Eden a little further down the road, at the next crossing, quickly becomes our main way of dealing with stress once again. Sadly, we often carry on like this till the day of our death.

Research on the benefits of cardiac coherence leads to a radically different conclusion: The problem has to be turned on its head. Instead of perpetually trying to produce ideal external circumstances, we must begin by controlling what is inside—our physiology. By reducing physiological chaos and maximizing coherence, we automatically feel better immediately. We improve our relations with others, our concentration, our performance, and our bottom line. Progressively, the ideal circumstances we are constantly seeking begin to come about on their own, but this phenomenon is almost a by-product, a secondary benefit of coherence. Once we have mastered our own inner being, what happens in the world outside has less of a grip on us. And we actually have a better grip on our world.

Software programs that measure coherence in cardiac rhythm are used for research on the heart-brain system, but they can also be used to demonstrate to anyone who doubts that one's heart would instantly react to one's emotional state. (See chapter 15 for more information on how you purchase such a software program yourself, or find someone who can help you use one.) However, it is perfectly possible to create coherence within the self without a computer and to immediately feel its benefits in everyday life. To do so, you simply learn how to live with heart coherence. This is the topic of the next chapter.

4

Living with Heart Coherence

In medical parlance, Ron was an "intensivist"—a specialist in intensive care—in the hospital where I was chief of the psychiatry department. He asked me to see a high-powered, 32-year-old management consultant who had had a myocardial infarction two days earlier. My colleague was worried about the seriousness of the young man's depression. He wanted me to examine him as soon as possible, because he knew from the scientific literature that patients who sink into depression after a heart attack have a poor prognosis. Moreover, the patient showed very low heart rate variability, an additional sign of how serious his condition was. Ron did not know what to recommend to deal with this second peril, nor to whom to turn. At that time, I did not know either.

Moreover, Ron's patient did not want to speak to a psychiatrist—as often happens with high-stress/high-power people. Although I had been told that his emotional life was painful, he rejected all my efforts to talk about the circumstances of his infarction or to discuss his troubles with me. He also remained evasive about his working conditions. He thought that stress was just part and parcel of his line of work and that his body should adjust to it. After all, his colleagues were subject to the same pressures and they had not had heart attacks. In any event, a psychiatrist who, unlike him, did *not* have a Harvard degree, was not going to tell him how to run his life.

Despite our strained conversation, I could see something frail and almost childlike in his face. I was also touched by the boundless ambition that had propelled him on since childhood and that was crushing him now, and his heart as well. There was something sensitive about him, perhaps even artistic—something that was struggling to emerge from behind that cold front. He left the hospital the next day, against his cardiologist's advice, and went back to his office, which "was waiting for him." I was sad to learn from Ron that he had died 6 months later of a second infarction, this time without even having had time to get to the hospital, just as he had not had time to open up to his own sensitivity. I was also sorry not to have known how to help him. Neither my colleague nor I knew then that there was a simple and effective method to increase heart rate variability and bring it into coherence, one that didn't demand that he seek any kind of long-term therapy.

The Coherence Training Method

Heart coherence was first described in 1992 by physicist Dan Winter and was made popular more recently by the Institute of HeartMath based in Boulder Creek, California. They developed and researched a number of techniques and practical applications of cardiac coherence. Their work has been developed further by others in Europe, such as Alan Watkins, M.D., Ph.D., based in London.

The practice of heart coherence draws together a number of ancient wisdoms and traditional techniques used in yoga, mindfulness, meditation, and relaxation. The first stage consists of turning your attention inward. To start with, you must set aside your personal concerns for a few minutes. You have to be willing to keep your worries briefly waiting and give your heart and brain the time it takes to recover their balance and intimacy.

The best way to go about this is to begin by taking two deep, slow breaths. They will immediately stimulate the parasympathetic system and begin applying a bit of physiological "brake." To maximize their effect, your attention must stay focused on your breath right up until you have finished exhaling and then let your breathing pause for a few seconds before the next in-breath begins of its own accord. The point is to let your mind float with the out-breath right up to the point where it lightens up, becoming mellow and buoyant inside your chest.

Eastern meditation practices would suggest concentrating on the breath as long as possible and keeping the mind empty. But to maximize cardiac coherence, it works better to actually center your attention on the region of your heart 10 to 15 seconds after your breathing stabilizes. At this second stage, imagine that you are breathing through your heart (or the center of your chest, if you do not yet feel your heart directly). As you continue breathing slowly and deeply (but effortlessly), visualize—and really feel—each inhalation and exhalation passing through that key part of your body. Imagine that each intake of oxygen nourishes your body and each exhalation rids it of the waste it no longer needs. Imagine the slow and supple movements of inhalation and exhalation that bathe the body in this purifying and soothing air. Imagine that they are helping your body make the most of the gift of attention and respite it is receiving from you. You might visualize your heart as a child in a bath of lukewarm water where it floats and frolics freely, at its own pace, without constraints or obligations. Like a beloved child at play, you ask her only to be herself. You watch her thriving in her natural element, as you continue to supply gentle and enveloping air.

The third stage consists in becoming aware of the sensation of warmth or expansiveness that is developing in your chest, and in fostering and encouraging it with your thoughts and your breath. This feeling is often shy at the beginning and emerges only discreetly. After years of emotional abuse, the heart is often like an animal awakening from long hibernation. First it feels the first warm whiffs of spring air. Numb and uncertain, it opens one eye, then two, and it only springs to action after making certain that the mild weather is not just a chance occurrence. One way to encourage the heart is to draw on a feeling of recognition or gratitude and to let it fill your chest. The heart is particularly sensitive to gratitude, to any feelings of love, whether it be love for another being, an object, or even the idea of a benevolent universe. To many, it is enough to think of the face of a beloved child, or even a pet. To others, a peaceful scene in nature brings on a sensation of inner gratitude. For you, maybe inner gratitude will spring from the memory of a physical feat—the exhilaration of a downhill ski run, the perfect swing of a golf club, or the hauling in of a sail as you lean into the wind. During this exercise, people sometimes notice a gentle smile that has risen to their lips, as if it had spread from the glow inside their chest. That is a simple sign that coherence has been established. Other signs include a sensation of lightness, warmth, or expansion in your chest.

In a study published by the *American Journal of Cardiology*, Dr. Watkins and researchers from the HeartMath Institute have demonstrated that the very act of recollecting a positive emotion or imagining a pleasurable scene rapidly provokes a transition of heart rate variability toward a phase of coherence.[2] Coherence in heart rhythm affects the emotional brain, fostering stability and signalling that everything is in working order physiologically. The emotional brain reacts to this message by reinforcing coherence in the heart. This interplay creates a "virtuous" circle that, with a little practice, may lead to a state of maximum coherence lasting for 30 minutes or more. Coherence between the heart and the emotional brain stabilizes the autonomic nervous system, both sympathetic and parasympathetic. Having reached a state of balance, we are optimally poised to confront any and all contingencies. We simultaneously have access to the wisdom of the emotional brain—its "intuition"—and to the faculties for reflection, abstract reasoning, and planning of the cognitive brain.

The more training we have in using this technique, the easier it becomes to induce coherence. Once accustomed to this inner state, we become capable of communicating directly, so to speak, with our heart. Like Celeste talking to the little fairy who lived in her heart, we can ask questions such as, "At the bottom of my heart, do I really love him/her?" and get a real answer.

Once coherence is established, we have only to ask ourselves the question and carefully observe our heart's reaction. If this reaction provokes an extra wave of inner warmth, of well-being, at the very least it wishes to maintain the contact. If, on the contrary, the heart seems to withdraw slightly—if coherence declines—it seeks avoidance and prefers focusing its energy elsewhere. This does not necessarily provide the right answer. After all, many couples go through periods where their hearts would like to be elsewhere, at least temporarily, before making up and rediscovering a lasting happiness in their relationship. Nevertheless, it is very important to be conscious of the heart's preference at each stage in life, because it has a powerful influence on the present. In this authentic inner dialogue, I imagine the heart as a sort of bridge to our "visceral self," acting on behalf of the emotional brain, suddenly open to a nearly direct form of communication. And we all need to find out if our emotional brain is pointing in a different direction from the one we have chosen rationally. If this is so, we must try to reassure the emotional brain in other ways, so as to avoid a conflict with our cognitive brain. Such a conflict would sabotage our capacities for reflection. In the end, it would produce physiological chaos and its ultimate consequence, a chronic waste of energy.

Different software programs exist that measure heart rate variability and let anyone visualize the impact of his or her thoughts on coherence and chaos at a second's notice. (See chapter 15 for more information on this software.) When you focus your attention on the heart and inner well-being, you can see the change in phase taking place and coherence taking over in the shape of gentle, regular waves. On the other hand, as soon as you let negative thoughts or worries divert your attention—which is the normal tendency of the brain left to its own devices—coherence diminishes in a few seconds and chaos takes over. If you yield to anger, chaos breaks out immediately, and the curve on the screen mimics a mountainous horizon that seems almost threatening in its spiky peaks. While biofeedback software in general has been available for many years, it has typically focused on measures of "relaxation" such as increased temperature in the fingers, decreased activity of sweat glands, or reduction of heart rate. With the discovery of the importance of heart rate variability, biofeedback systems focused on coherence are just now starting to become widely available to help speed up training.

Still, even before computers, we have had ways to establish coherence. I have often observed that my patients or acquaintances who practice yoga can induce coherence easily when I test them with a computer. Their physiology seemed to have already been partially transformed by their regular exercises.

In the same vein, too much focus on the technical aspects of the method can be a hindrance. When I demonstrated this method to a friend who has a deep spiritual life, he had trouble attaining more than 35 percent optimal coherence. He then asked me if he could simply pray as he usually does instead of following my instructions. As he prayed, he very quickly started to experience a warmth and well-being in his chest that seemed to correspond to what I had described. In a few moments, his coherence had risen to 80 percent. Clearly, my friend had found his own way of balancing his physiology, by immersing in his feeling of connectedness to an all-powerful and benevolent universe. However, prayer does not necessarily foster coherence in

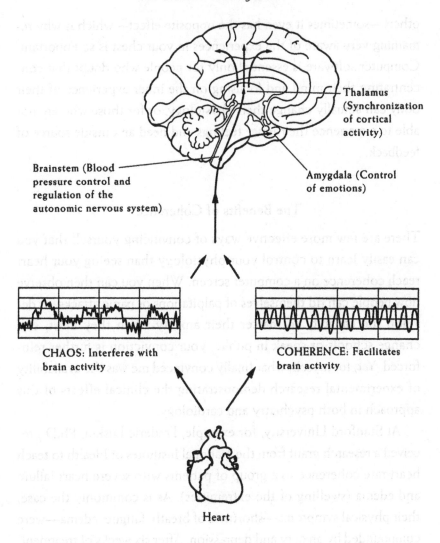

Thalamus
(Synchronization
of cortical
activity)

Brainstem (Blood
pressure control and
regulation of the
autonomic nervous system)

Amygdala (Control
of emotions)

CHAOS: Interferes with
brain activity

COHERENCE: Facilitates
brain activity

Heart

THE HEART HELPS THE BRAIN TO FUNCTION

According to some preliminary studies, the coherence of cardiac rhythm directly affects the brain's performance. Phases of chaos are thought to interfere with the synchronization of operations in the brain, whereas coherence contributes to their coordination. This results in faster and more accurate responses and better performance under stress. (Graph based on a presentation by Rollin McCraty, Research Director of the HeartMath Institute in Boulder Creek, California.)

others—sometimes it even has the opposite effect—which is why remaining very aware of the experiences in your chest is so important. Computer software is essential only for people who doubt that concentrating their mind and focusing on the inner experience of their body can actually change their physiology, or for those who are not able to experience their inner feelings and need an outside source of feedback.

The Benefits of Coherence

There are few more effective ways of convincing yourself that you can easily learn to control your physiology than seeing your heart reach coherence on a computer screen. When you can then observe how people can rid themselves of palpitations or panic attacks, or develop the capacity to master their anxiety when they must, say, change schools or speak in public, your conviction is further reinforced. Yet, for myself, what finally convinced me was the availability of experimental research demonstrating the clinical effects of this approach in both psychiatry and cardiology.

At Stanford University, for example, Frederic Luskin, Ph.D., received a research grant from the National Institutes of Health to teach heart rate coherence to a group of patients with severe heart failure and edema (swelling of the extremities). As is commonly the case, their physical symptoms—shortness of breath, fatigue, edema—were compounded by anxiety and depression. After six weeks of treatment, the group that had learned to master heart coherence had considerably lowered its stress (by 22 percent) and depression (by 34 percent). The physical status of the patients in that group—their capacity to walk without getting out of breath—had distinctly improved (by 14 percent). These results contrasted sharply with the control group, which had received conventional treatment for heart failure. Compared with their starting point, all of their symptoms had worsened.[3]

In London, 6,000 executives from major corporations such as Shell, British Petroleum, Hewlett Packard, Unilever, and the Hong Kong Shanghai Bank Corporation followed a training course in heart rate coherence. In the United States, several thousand others have been trained at the HeartMath Institute, among them the staff of Motorola and government employees of the state of California. Follow-up testing of these participants shows that their training counteracted stress from three different standpoints—physical, emotional, and social.

A month after training, the data on the training's physical impact on participants was striking. It suggested that the drop in their blood pressure was the same as could have been expected after a 20-pound weight loss, and twice as great as it would have been after following a salt-free diet.[4] Another study suggests a distinct improvement in hormone balance. After 1 month's practice of coherence for 30 minutes a day, 5 days a week, the percentage of DHEA (dehydroepiandrosterone)—the so-called "youth" hormone[5]—doubled. With these same subjects, the percentage of cortisol—the quintessential stress hormone, associated with increases in blood pressure, skin aging, and loss of memory and concentration[6]—had declined by 23 percent.[7] The women observed in this study displayed a distinct improvement in their premenstrual symptoms, with less irritability, depression, and fatigue. Such hormone changes reflect a profound restoration of the body's physiological balance, which is all the more striking because it occurs without medication or synthetic hormones.

The immune system also appears to benefit from the practice of cardiac coherence. Immunoglobulin A (IgA) represents the body's front line of defense against infectious agents (viruses, bacteria, and fungi). IgA is constantly renewed on the surface of mucous membranes such as the nose, the throat, the lungs' bronchi, the intestines, and the vagina—all sites where infections are a permanent threat. Volunteers in an experiment were asked to think about a scene they had lived through in which they had become angry. The simple recollection of this event led to several minutes of chaos in their cardiac rhythm. After that period of chaos, the secretion of IgA dropped for an average of 6 hours, thereby lowering their resistance to infection. The same experiment showed that recollecting a positive memory, which triggered several minutes of coherence, resulted in an *increase* in the production of IGA for the next 6 hours.*[8] In another study, published more than 10 years ago in the *New England Journal of Medicine*, researchers in Pittsburgh demonstrated that subjects' stress level directly affects their likelihood of catching a cold.

The greater the stress, the more likely subjects were to become clinically ill.[9] This phenomenon may well be due to the effect of negative emotions on the heart-brain system and the immune system. Every time we have an unpleasant altercation at the office, or with our spouse, or even in the street, our line of defense against infections lowers its guard for 6 hours! Unless, it seems, we succeed in maintaining our coherence.

Research on corporate managers shows how learning to induce coherence can lead to a substantial decline in the usual symptoms of stress. The number of executives who say they have palpitations "often or almost all the time" falls from 47 percent—an astounding figure—to 30 percent after 6 weeks, and to 25 percent after 3 months. Symptoms of physical tension drop from 41 percent to 15 percent, then to 6 percent. Insomnia declines from 34 percent to 6 percent, feelings of exhaustion from 50 percent to 12 percent, different aches and pains—including backache—from 30 percent to 6 percent. According to several of these corporate participants, mental fatigue had become a "normal" feature of their work, the way physical fatigue was considered normal in the mines and factories at

---

*In a comparable study, the well-known mindfulness meditation clinical program of the University of Massachusetts Medical School, developed by Jon Kabat-Zinn, Ph.D., was used with employees of a biotechnology corporation. Following the 8-week training, those in the meditation group had a significant rise in antibody titers that correlated with the degree to which they increased positive affect in their brain, as measured by EEG (electroencephalogram). (Davidson, J. K. T., J. Kabat-Zinn, et al., "Alternations in Brain and Immune Function Produced by Mindfulness Meditation," *Psychosomatic Medicine* 65 (2003): 564–570.)

the start of the industrial revolution. After they learned to gear their physiological responses to the constant demands of their work, these executives trained in coherence would say that they now knew how to reduce the constant leaking of their energy.

In the psychological domain, the figures are equally striking. The proportion of employees who say they are "anxious" most of the time in large corporations declines from 33 percent (one out of three!) to 5 percent. Those who say they are "dissatisfied," from 30 percent to 9 percent; those who declare they are "angry" from 20 percent to 8 percent. Participants describe a new ability to handle their feelings. They say that practicing coherence has made them realize that episodes of anger and negative feelings are useless and that workdays in the office are a lot more pleasant without such occurrences.

Charles, whose story we encountered in the preceding chapter, recognizes himself in these figures. Yet the transition took place little by little. When he recalls how he took everything "to heart" before training in coherence, he wonders how he could have gone on for so long. He remembers the state in which the president's remarks used to leave him, sometimes for hours. How incapable he was of ridding himself of these feelings, even at home at night when, sleepless, he tossed and turned in bed, sometimes for weeks at a time. He now feels calmer, capable of letting such remarks "glide" over him. After all, the president talked to everyone like that—it was the sort of man he was. That was *his* problem, not Charles's. Charles had learned to calm his physiology, to stop it from getting carried away. In fact, his doctor was surprised to notice a reduction in his blood pressure. He asked him if he had gone on a diet without telling him.

When it comes to company operations and social relations, groups that have learned to master their inner responses work more harmoniously. In corporations that were tested in the United Kingdom 6 weeks and 6 months after training in coherence, executives said they were thinking more clearly, listening to each other more, and holding more productive meetings. In a major hospital in the Chicago area where nurses had been trained, their job satisfaction had distinctly improved. At the same time, their patients said they were better satisfied with the nursing care they received. The turnover in nurses in the year following their training fell from 20 percent to 4 percent.[10] Finally, a study carried out on American high school students shows to what extent effective management of an individual's inner state can change performance under stress. These students had repeated a class after failing to graduate. After training in coherence for 2 hours a week over 8 weeks, 64 percent of the students passed the mathematics exam, compared to only 42 percent of those who had not received this training. Obviously, coherence does not change mathematical knowledge, but it makes existing knowledge more readily accessible when taking a stressful test.[11]

Living in Coherence

Françoise Dolto, M.D., an outstanding child psychiatrist in France in the 1970s, knew better than anyone else how to talk to children who were in emotional pain. With a lost child who was incapable of explaining what was hurting and who was thus inconsolable, she would start out by asking a magic question: "What does your heart feel?" She knew that with these few words she was opening the door directly on emotions, cutting through a jumble of mental constructions, of "I should"s or "I shouldn't"s. She helped those suffering to get in touch with their inner workings, their profound desires, the very things that, in the final analysis, determine well-being or unhappiness.

The same is true for adults—especially for the most rational among us, those who tend to perceive and react only through the intermediary of their cognitive brains. A whole unknown world of sensations and emotions opens up to them when they look in on their heart's reactions. Once coherence is established, they often realize that their inner intuitive self has been guiding them all along, and they feel

compassion, almost tenderness, for their inner being. As Eastern spiritual traditions suggest, that compassion for the inner being breeds
compassion for the outside world. Knowledge is within you. The act
of becoming aware of this makes you more open to others.

I often call on this intuition of the heart myself. I remember, for example, a difficult case of a young African-American patient who was in
great physical pain, but whose thorough examination and test results
did not reveal anything abnormal. After a few days, the doctors refused
to do any further testing. The patient wanted her doctors to give her
morphine, which the team refused to do, as there was no clear diagnosis. In tense circumstances like these it was not unusual for my colleagues to wind up calling in a psychiatrist. The young woman was
furious at the suggestion that her problems were "all in her head." She
agreed to see me only in the presence of her mother, who was even
more determined to get additional tests. From their point of view, the
doctors' refusal to carry out further examinations was a clear proof of
racism. If the hospital was refusing to do more, it was because she was
neither white nor rich.

My day had been long and difficult. When they greeted me with
a volley of insults, without giving me time to introduce myself, I felt
a sense of irritation welling up that bordered on anger. I walked out of
the room abruptly. In the corridor I realized that I felt flushed and
even spiteful. Like a teacher who has been jeered at by a pupil, I began
to think of all the trouble I could make for them to make them pay for
their "bad behavior." Observing this inner state, I began by taking two
deep breaths and let myself enter into coherence, focusing my attention on my heart, and then thinking of fishing for winkles with my son
at sunset in Normandy. Once calm was restored and my mind perfectly clear, I thought about the situation once more. New ideas
seemed to spring forth from another part of myself. Clearly this young
woman must have greatly suffered if she felt such rage against people
who were doing their best to help her. She must have been rejected

and misunderstood a number of times. And my attitude could not have helped her change her opinion of the hospital doctors, almost all of whom were white. Wasn't it my job, after all, to know how to help people with difficult personalities? If I, as a psychiatrist, could not succeed in communicating with her, who else could? And how could I have had such childish thoughts of "revenge?" What a lot of good that would have done!

Suddenly, I thought of a new way to approach her. I ought to go back into the room and tell her, "You have the right to the best care possible from my colleagues and from me. I am truly sorry if we haven't lived up to your expectations. If you are willing, I would now like to find out what has been going on here and how we have disappointed you." Once the conversation got started, I would probably find out enough to grasp the real cause of her suffering. Perhaps I would then be able to suggest a more effective approach than the additional tests, which would be as unpleasant to her as they were unnecessary. What did I have to lose? I went back into the room in that new state of mind and made my offer. Their hostile looks gradually brightened. We got into a real conversation. I found out how several emergency services had sent the young woman away, how a doctor had insulted her, and, little by little, the conversation became more intimate. She finally asked her mother to leave the room. Then we were able to talk about her past as a prostitute and her experience as a drug addict. Some of her present pain was simply due to heroin withdrawal symptoms. That was something that could be handled easily. I promised to help her reduce the pain caused by withdrawal, and we left each other on excellent terms. She was confident that she was finally going to be helped, and I was happy to have been able to do my job as a doctor. As I left her room for the second time, I shuddered as I thought about how close I had come, out of anger, to having her sent home without further treatment.

During her divorce, Christine, who had also learned to induce inner coherence, experienced a very similar situation with her son

Thomas, who was 5. She had offered to take him to the zoo on a Saturday morning, but he was not making any effort to find his shoes. She was in a hurry and in her head she heard the voice of her best friend saying, "If you don't deal with your son's messiness now, it will only get worse. Wait until he gets to be an adolescent!" Christine started to scold her child for his chronic incapacity to pick up his things, which always ended up making them late. Thomas's reaction was to sit down on the floor, cross his arms, and act like a misunderstood, martyred child about to burst out crying. It was the last straw. Christine, who was tense because of the family situation, decided to leave without him and leave him with her mother, who had come in to help for the day. She was determined not to be taken in once again by her son's emotional manipulations.

Once in her car, she took stock of her inner feelings. She was still angry and tense, even more so now that she realized that the rest of the day and, probably, the rest of the weekend, were going to be spoiled by this catastrophic beginning. She started to apply her training in coherence and, as soon as inner calm began to take hold, another perspective opened up to her. What if Thomas's lateness and disorganization this morning were not caused by his usual untidiness? What if they resulted from his distress about his parents' divorce? She saw herself in his place for a moment, as a confused 5-year-old child, incapable of expressing her fear and unhappiness. She also imagined how she would have reacted in such circumstances if her mother had not understood her and had persisted in making a fuss about something as trivial as not putting her shoes on. What kind of example was she setting for her son? Did she want him to learn to handle emotional tensions by storming out of the room and slamming the door as, in fact, she had just done?

Suddenly she saw clearly that she had to take the risk of "losing face" and going home to talk to Thomas. "I'm sorry to have gotten so upset," she told him. "After all, the zoo isn't all that important. What's important is that you are a little sad and that it's normal in the situation you and your father and I are in. And when people are sad, they often have trouble picking up their things. I'm sad, too, and that's why I get upset too easily. But if you and I are aware of this, it will be easier for us to work things out."

Thomas looked up and burst into tears. Christine took him in her arms and hugged him. A little while later he was smiling again and they spent a fine day together. In fact, Thomas was more organized and attentive than ever. Once emotional energy is freed by coherence, we can often find the answers, as well as the words, that reconcile rather than separate. And when we do, we stop wasting energy.

Coherence leads to inner calm, but it is not a relaxation technique. It is meant to facilitate action. Coherence can be practiced in any everyday situation. You can establish coherence just as well when your heart rate is 120 as when it is 55 beats a minute. That is actually the ultimate goal: to maintain coherence during the excitement of a race or a fight, when facing the pain of defeat, but also in the pleasure of victory and even in ecstasy. Handbooks on Eastern sexuality teach that focusing the mind on the heart helps to master and maximize pleasure. Tantric and Taoist masters had probably grasped, long before computer software was available, the positive effect of cardiac coherence during intercourse.

The results experienced by men and women who have discovered coherence and practice it regularly are almost too good to be true. The control of anxiety and depression, the lowering of blood pressure, the increase in the hormone DHEA (dehydroepiandrosterone), the stimulation of the immune system—what these preliminary results suggest is not only a slowing down of the aging process, but a turning back of the physiological clock. However difficult to believe, the nature of these results matches the nature of the physical and psychological damage inflicted by stress. If stress can cause so much harm, I am not entirely surprised that inner mastery can do so much good.

However, for those of us who have been wounded by life and whose scars are not yet healed, it may be painful and anxiety provoking to look inward. In this case, access to our inner source of coherence may be blocked. Usually this happens as a result of a trauma in which emotions have been so overwhelming that the emotional brain, and thus the heart, no longer operates the same way. The heart-mind system is no longer a compass but a flag fluttering in the wind. In this case, another approach can recover balance, a method as surprising as it is effective, which may have its origin in the mechanism of dreams: eye movement desensitization and reprocessing.

5

Eye Movement Desensitization and Reprocessing (EMDR): The Mind's Own Healing Mechanism

After a year of idyll, Mark, the man whom Sarah was sure she would marry, had left her without warning. There hadn't been a single cloud on their relationship. Their bodies had seemed to be made for each other and their vivacious minds—they were both lawyers—were in agreement on everything. She loved so many things about Mark: his voice, his smell, his laugh that roared constantly. She even liked her future in-laws. All their plans were drawn. But, one day, Mark knocked on her door with an orange tree in his arms dressed with a large ribbon. In his hands, he was holding a letter that told her what he could not say with his own voice. The words were cold and harsh. He had gotten back with his former girlfriend, who was Catholic, like him, and she would be the woman whom he would marry. His decision was final, the letter said.

The Scar in the Brain

After that afternoon, Sarah was never the same. She had always been a rock, but she started to have anxiety attacks at the slightest reminder of what had happened to her. She could no longer sit next to a small indoor tree, especially not an orange tree. Her heart would beat in her chest any time she would hold an envelope with her name handwritten on it. Sometimes, for no apparent reason, she would have flashbacks: She would see the scene of Mark's departure right in front of her eyes, as if it were happening all over again. At night, she would sometimes dream of Mark and wake up with a start. She wouldn't dress the same way anymore, she would not walk the same way, not smile the same way. For a long time, she would be unable to talk about what had happened to her, overcome with a mixture of shame—how could she have been so wrong about Mark?—and embarrassment, because tears would well up as soon as she would recall the memory. Talking about it was impossible; she could hardly create a sentence to describe what had happened to her. The few words that would come up seemed so insufficient, so lame.

As the story of Sarah illustrates—and as we all know from our own experiences—traumatic events leave marks in our brains. A study from the department of psychiatry at Harvard Medical School showed what this mark in the brain might look like. People who had experienced a severe trauma—"posttraumatic stress disorder," or PTSD—were listening to a tape recounting the incident while lying in a PET (positron emission topography) scanner. The scanner images showed which parts of their brains were activated or inactivated during these minutes of reexperienced terror, and there was a clear activation of the amygdala and surrounding region: the center for fear in the emotional brain. The subjects' visual cortex was also activated, almost as if they were looking at a photograph of the event right in front of their eyes. And even more fascinating was a "deactivation"—a sort of anesthesia—of Broca's area in the left prefrontal cortex, the brain's region responsible for the expression of language. The PET scanner was showing us the neurological signature of what we so often hear patients say. "There are no words to describe what I went through."[1]

Psychiatrists know that these scars in the brain are hard to erase. People often continue to experience symptoms decades after the original trauma. This phenomenon is commonly seen in Vietnam veterans or in survivors of the Holocaust, but it is also true of traumas that occur in civilian life. A study found that a *majority* of women with PTSD who had been victims of an aggression still suffered from the condition 10 years later.[2] What is fascinating, of course, is that most of these people know perfectly well that they should no longer be feeling this way. They know that the Vietnam War is over, the Holocaust a nightmare from the past, or the rape a distant memory. They *know* that they are safe now, but they do not *feel* this way.

The Lasting Trace of Pain

We can all understand this from our own experience, because, in fact, most of us have experienced what may be called "small-t" traumas, as opposed to the "big-T" trauma of life-threatening experiences usually associated with a diagnosis of PTSD. We may have been humiliated in grade school, been rejected harshly by a boyfriend or girlfriend, or made a serious mistake in our professional life, perhaps lost our job abruptly. It may even have been a difficult divorce that left us emotionally scarred. Undoubtedly, we have thought about it quite a bit on our own, received a lot of advice from friends and family, read magazine articles about this type of situation and how to respond to it, perhaps even read self-help books. From all of these sources, we learned, often very well, how to *think* about the situation, and we know how we *should* be feeling about it. However, this is often where things are left: with feelings that have lagged behind and remain anchored in the past even after our rational (cognitive) understanding has changed. The man who had a car accident continues to feel uncomfortable and tense when he drives on the highway, even though he knows full well that the accident was not his fault and that he drove for years on the same highway without problems. The woman who was sexually assaulted continues to freeze when attempting to become physically intimate with a man she loves, even though she is very clear about her affection for him and her desire for intimacy. It is as if the neural networks in the cognitive brain that represent all the appropriate cognitions have not linked up with the neural networks in the emotional brain that continue to encode the painful emotions.[3]

In a laboratory at New York University, a researcher born in Louisiana has shed new light on the way these emotional traces are organized in the brain. As a child, Joseph LeDoux, Ph.D., watched his father, a butcher, cutting up cattle brains. To this day, he is still fascinated by the structure of that organ. After years spent studying the difference between the left and right brains, Dr. LeDoux wanted to understand how the emotional and cognitive brains relate to each other. He was one of the first researchers to demonstrate that fear reactions are not encoded in the neocortex. He discovered that when an animal learns to be afraid of something, the memory trace is formed directly in the emotional brain.[4]

In these studies, rats are placed in a cage with electric flooring. Whenever a bell rings, they receive small shocks through their paws. After a few bell rings and shocks, rats quickly learn to freeze in fear whenever the bell comes on. If the experiment stops for a while, the rats' fear response persists, even months later when they again hear the bell (or any other sound similar to it). However, it is possible to do "therapy" with these rats by ringing the bell repeatedly and *not* shocking them. This "exposure therapy," a form of behavior therapy, is well-known to "extinguish" the fear response. After enough exposure of this kind, it looks as if the rats learn that the bell is no longer to be feared since it no longer predicts the onset of the electric shock. Even when the bell goes off, they just go about their usual activities. This finding, one of the oldest results of the classical conditioning literature, has been known since Pavlov as "extinction" of the fear response through "exposure."[5] For all practical purposes, it looks as if the trace of the fear response has been erased from the rats' emotional brains. However, the reality is much different.

Dr. LeDoux, and other scientists who have worked with him, such as Greg Quirk, Ph.D., now at the Ponce School of Medicine, have found that the trace in the emotional brain never completely disappears. Rats behave "as if" they have no fear only as long as the prefrontal cortex is actively blocking the automatic response of the emotional brain. As soon as the control of the neocortex weakens, fear takes over again, even after the "therapy."[6] Dr. LeDoux also talks about the "indelibility" of emotional memories.[7] The "exposure therapy," with which the rats seem to do better initially, seems to leave the fear response of the emotional brain untouched, ready to be reactivated. Extrapolating to human patients, these results in animals help us understand how scars in the emotional brain may last for decades, ready and waiting to manifest again.

I met Paulina when she was 60 years old. She was seeking help because she felt irrationally uncomfortable in the presence of her new boss. Two weeks earlier, as he stood behind her in her office, she had broken into an uncontrollable sweat and she hadn't been able to continue her phone conversation with an important client. Ten years before, she had already lost a job because of a similar problem. Now she was determined to do something about it.

I quickly found out that she'd had an alcoholic and violent father. He had beaten her on several occasions when she was a child. I asked her to describe one of the worst scenes. She told me how, when she was 5 years old, her father had come home with a brand new car and seemed to be in a particularly good mood. She had wanted to take advantage of this to get closer to him. When he went into the house, she thought that, to make him happy, she could make the car shine even more by cleaning it. She found a bucket and a sponge and she started rubbing it with all the enthusiasm of a little girl who wanted to please her father. Unfortunately, she had not noticed that there was some gravel left in the bucket and which stuck to the sponge. When her father came outside to see the car, he saw that it had been scratched from one end to the other, and on both sides. A rage came over him that seemed completely incomprehensible to the little girl. Scared of what he might do, she ran upstairs to her room and hid under her bed. Thinking about that memory brought back the image that seemed to have been imprinted into her brain as clearly as a photograph: the feet of her father coming toward her while she crouched under the bed, as close as possible to the wall, like a small animal.

Together with that picture, the emotion of that moment was coming back with its full power. In front of me, 55 years later, I could see her face deformed by fear. Her breathing was fast, all her muscles seemed tense, and I remember being afraid that she might have a heart attack in my office. Fifty-five years later, her entire brain, her entire body could be thrown into fear by the scar of that event.

After the rats have learned to fear a bell that warns them of a shock, they freeze whenever any bell rings that resembles that original sound.[8] In the case of Paulina, it was enough for her boss to look even vaguely like her father to make her acutely uncomfortable, even many years later.

It seems that the scars in our emotional brain remain ready to express themselves whenever the cognitive brain and the power of reason lower their vigilance: when we drink alcohol, for example, take mind-altering drugs, are excessively tired, or are too distracted by other preoccupations to maintain control over the limbic fear. These conditions demonstrate a true "disconnect" between the cognitive and the emotional brain after traumatic events have left a deep scar: Both parts of the brain are pulling in different directions rather than finding a way to integrate the past and the present in a harmonious pattern.

The Eye Movements of Dreams

Psychiatrists know about this "disconnect" with PTSD. They realize that this detachment between the appropriate thoughts and the inappropriate leftover emotions from the trauma is precisely what makes it so hard to treat. They know that just talking about the trauma often fails to produce the necessary connection between the old emotional memory and a more appropriate view grounded in the present. In fact, they know that simply remembering the trauma often seems to make people worse rather than better.

Psychiatrists also know that medications only have limited effectiveness. In the early 1990s, a review of treatments for posttraumatic stress disorder published in the prestigious *Journal of the American Medical Association* concluded that there were no truly effective treatments for this condition, only interventions with limited benefits.[9] In my experience with patients, I was keenly aware of this fact. Like my colleagues, I had struggled to help victims of emotional trauma for years with only limited success, until one day, I saw a remarkable videotape.

Francine Shapiro, Ph.D., a senior research fellow at the Mental Research Institute of Palo Alto, who discovered Eye Movement Desensitization and Reprocessing (EMDR), was presenting her method at a behavioral medicine meeting I was attending. I had heard of EMDR and was extremely skeptical that making people move their eyes back and forth in imitation of the rapid eye movements that take place during dreams could do anything to help heal trauma. However, one of the cases caught my attention.

Maggie, a woman in her sixties, had been diagnosed with an aggressive throat cancer and her doctor had told her that she had 6 months to live and that she would die a slow and painful death. Her husband of 27 years was a widower from a previous marriage, and as fate would have it, his previous wife had died of cancer. When Maggie told him of the doctor's verdict, Henry felt so overwhelmed that he said he just could not go through that again. And then, he left her.

Maggie was in shock and became profoundly depressed. She bought a gun with the intention of killing herself. Learning of this, friends convinced Henry to come back and stay with her again. However, Maggie had been so traumatized by Henry's abandonment that she could not sleep, was having recurrent nightmares of him leaving again, and could not tolerate being separated from him even for the purpose of grocery shopping. Hearing of a study to help people recover from trauma, she participated in one of the early controlled studies of EMDR.

At first, she could not even evoke the image of Henry backing out of the driveway on the day of his departure. She would immediately almost suffocate with fear. Then, with the help of a caring and attentive therapist, she was able to let herself recall the most painful images of Henry leaving while she followed her therapist's hand, moving back and forth in front of her eyes. Talking about her pain clearly took an enormous effort, and the memory seemed to be encoded primarily throughout her body. She would complain not only of fear but of her heart pounding and of "hurting all over."

Then, all of a sudden, after another set of eye movements, Maggie's face changed completely. She had a surprised expression on her face, and she said, "It's gone!"

"It's like I was on a train," she recalled. "You look at something that seems completely there for a moment, and then it's gone; it's in the past and there's something else instead you're looking at. Whether it was beauty or pain, it's in the past. You can't recapture that."

Her entire body language was different. She now looked composed, though still somewhat dazzled. With the next set of eye movements, she started smiling. The therapist stopped the eye movements and asked her what had come to her mind. She said, "I have something funny to tell you. I just saw myself standing on the porch and looking at Henry in the driveway and I thought, 'If he can't deal with this, that's his problem, not mine.' I was waving at him and saying, 'Bye, Henry, bye.' Can you believe that? 'Bye, Henry, bye. . . . '"

As the session continued, with more brief series of eye movements, Maggie started talking spontaneously, or "free-associating," to the scene of her deathbed. She could see friends there and she knew that she would not be alone. At the end of the next series of eye movements, instead of the fear with which she had started the session, her face showed a new expression of resolution. She slapped her hand on her lap and said, "And you know what? I'm going to die with dignity!" The whole treatment had lasted perhaps 15 minutes, and the therapist had barely said 10 sentences.

The scientist part of me kept whispering, "This is just one patient . . . maybe she's particularly suggestible . . . maybe this is all a placebo effect." However, if this was a placebo effect, I decided that I definitely wanted to learn how to induce placebo effects like this in my own patients. I had simply never seen anything like that happen before.

What finally convinced me was a study of 80 patients with emotional trauma who were treated with EMDR, which was published in one of the most demanding journals in clinical psychology, the *Journal of Consulting and Clinical Psychology*. In that study, 80 percent of patients experienced a recovery from their traumatic syndromes within three 90-minute sessions.[10] This recovery rate is comparable to that of antibiotics in pneumonia.[11] I don't know of any treatment in psychiatry, including the most powerful medications, that has ever reported results of this magnitude over 3 weeks.

Of course, I worried that results achieved so rapidly could not possibly last. However, the same group of patients had been followed for 15 months and found to have exactly the same benefits 15 months after the treatment as at the end of the three sessions. Given such data, I thought it would be unconscionable for me *not* to learn EMDR and see for myself.

Self-Healing Mechanisms in the Brain

EMDR starts with the idea of an "adaptive information-processing system" that is built into our nervous system to help us grow psychologically. The concept is simple: We all experience "small-t" traumas throughout our lives. However, we generally don't develop PTSD. Say, for example, you had a bicycle accident: You were riding along a lane of parked cars, and someone suddenly opened his door right in front of you, too late for you to brake. In addition to the inevitable physical bruises, you may be bruised emotionally as well.

For a few hours, perhaps a few days, you may feel shaken in your body, you may think about the accident at unexpected times, talk about it frequently, dream about it at night. The next day, you may be nervous about getting on your bicycle again and, if you do, find yourself very vigilant about parked cars. However, within a short time, not long after your physical bruises are gone, you would most likely find yourself able to ride again. You would now pay more attention to parked cars and perhaps have learned to ride at a safe distance. In essence, you would have "digested" the painful event. Very much like the digestive system extracts from food what is useful and necessary for the body and rejects the waste, your nervous system would have extracted the useful information—the "lesson"—and discarded the emotions, thoughts, and physical arousal that are no longer necessary after the event is over.[12]

This psychological digestion process is what Freud described as "grief work" in his classic paper *Mourning and Melancholia*. After a serious loss, or any important challenge to our sense of safety in the world, our nervous system is temporarily disorganized and progressively finds its balance again (its "homeostasis," as physiologists say). Generally, it even grows stronger from this process, more flexible, more adaptive to a wider range of situations. Some psychiatrists have argued convincingly that it is precisely this process that helps us develop more resilience against adversity.[13] (Freud was writing when the industrial age was in full development and he referred to this phenomenon as the "work" of grieving. EMDR was developed during the computer revolution and the age of neuroscience; it refers to this digestion mechanism built into our brain as the "adaptive information-processing system.")

In some circumstances, however, our system's capacity to adapt can be overwhelmed. One is when the trauma is too strong, such as torture, rape, or the loss of a child (in my experience, the loss of a child, or even simply a child's serious illness, can be one of the most painful experiences people have to endure, and one of the hardest from which to recover). A second critical circumstance is when a trauma—even a much lesser one—takes place at a time when we are particularly vulnerable. Perhaps this event takes place in childhood, when we are physically powerless to defend ourselves and when our nervous system is not fully developed. It can also happen in adulthood if we were made fragile, physically or emotionally, for any reason. In either case—intense trauma or fragile victim—adverse events then become "traumatic," in the proper sense of the term.

Vera, for example, was a nurse who was consulting for chronic feelings of depression and a very low self-image. She thought of herself as "fat and ugly"—"disgusting," she would even say—whereas, objectively, she was rather attractive and her weight was well within the usual range. As she was also naturally fun and engaging, her self-image was clearly very distorted. While listening to her, I understood that this image of her body had taken root during the last few months of her pregnancy, several years before.

Vera distinctly remembered the day when she was arguing with her boyfriend, the father of the child. She was complaining that he wouldn't spend any time with her anymore. He had said he was "too busy," but she knew he was lying and she kept pushing him. He finally relented and shouted the "real" reason he was avoiding her: "You're so fat, you're the ugliest thing I've ever seen!"

Vera couldn't control her tears when she recalled this. "I thought I'd gotten over that," she started telling me. In other circumstances, she might well have been able to brush off her boyfriend's comment with her habitual wit. Perhaps she would have told him that he wasn't exactly Brad Pitt himself. But her pregnancy had been difficult; she had stopped working early on, and she wasn't sure she could find a job again when she went back. She was afraid that Jack might leave her right after the birth, just like her own father had left her mother. She felt powerless and vulnerable. The combination was enough for this toxic comment to take on a traumatizing dimension that it never should have had.

The Body's Memory of Emotions

As in the observations of the former director of the Harvard Psychological Trauma Clinic, the neuroscientist and psychiatrist Bessel van der Kolk, M.D., Ph.D., EMDR assumes that a trauma memory is information about the event that has become locked in the nervous system almost in its original form.[14] The images, thoughts, sounds, smells, emotions, physical sensations, and beliefs that instantly developed about the self (such as, "I'm powerless") are all stored together in a neural network that takes on its own life. Grounded in the emotional brain and disconnected from our rational knowledge about the world, that network becomes a packet of unprocessed and dysfunctional information that can become reactivated at the slightest reminder of the original trauma.

A memory in the brain can be accessed from any of its constituents; this is the so-called "content-addressable" property of the brain's memory system.[15] Just a whiff of perfume from a former lover can be enough for the entire memory of that person to come back: images, thoughts, and words. Furthermore, unlike computers that need exact matches, memory retrieval in the nervous system proceeds by analogy, so anything that even vaguely reminds us of something we know can bring back the memory. This trait has important consequences for traumatic memories. It means that any picture, sound, smell, emotion, thought, or even physical sensation that resembles what happened at the time of the event can bring back the entire experience of a dysfunctionally stored memory.

I have seen this function in dramatic form as a psychiatrist working in a general hospital. I was called to see a young woman who had just been brought out of the operating room. She was a little confused from the general anesthesia and had seemed agitated. The nurses were worried that in her confusion, she might pull on the tubes and IV lines that were still in place in her body. To prevent her from doing this, they had tied her wrists to her gurney with soft restraints. Shortly after, the woman had become wide awake and was screaming with an expression of terror on her face. She was fighting the restraints with all her strength, and her heart rate and blood pressure were shooting up, putting her at significant risk of an immediate medical complication. After I was able to calm her down (which involved removing the restraints), she described how she had just relived the memory of her stepfather tying her to her bed as a child and burning her skin with cigarette butts. The full memory, stored in its vivid, dysfunctional form, had been accessed from the sensation in her wrists.[16]

The thrust of EMDR is to evoke the traumatic memory in all of its different components—visual, emotional, cognitive, and, most of all, physical (the echo of the image in the body), and to then ask the patient to simply follow the hand of the therapist moving rapidly back and forth in front of his or her face in order to induce the appropriate eye movements. This process then stimulates the inborn "adaptive information-processing system" that has not been successful in metabolizing the dysfunctional memory by itself.

The idea is that inducing eye movements similar to that of REM (rapid eye movement) sleep provides a necessary assistance to the natural healing system of the mind that, so far, has not succeeded on its own. Just as certain plants and other natural remedies have been used for centuries to help the natural healing process of wounds from physical trauma, the eye movements of EMDR seem to accelerate the natural recovery from psychological trauma.

During the eye movements themselves, patients seem to be spontaneously free-associating through the vast network of related memories at different levels of consciousness. They frequently start seeing other scenes related to the same trauma, either because they were similar in nature (for example, another breakup, perhaps an earlier one), or because they shared a similar emotion (for example, being locked in a trunk as a 4-year-old by an older cousin). Or they may simply experience powerful emotions that quickly rise to the surface, even though they had been contained until then. It is as if the eye movements of EMDR facilitate rapid access to all the channels of association to the traumatic memory that's being targeted by the treatment. As these channels are evoked, they seem to rapidly link up with cognitive networks that store more appropriate information grounded in the present. It is through this connection that the perspective of the adult—who is no longer powerless, nor the prey of threats that belong to the past—can become anchored in the emotional brain. This new perspective can then replace the neurological imprint of fear or despair. And once this imprint has been replaced, it often seems as if a whole new person is allowed to emerge.

After several years of practicing EMDR, I remain surprised by the results that I continue to witness. I understand completely that many of my colleagues, psychiatrists or therapists, continue to be skeptical, just as I was myself for a long time. Yet, I know that I have not seen many treatments in medicine as intriguing as those when EMDR is put into action.

6

EMDR in Action

Lilian was an actress and drama teacher in a nationally renowned theater. She had acted all over the world, and she knew everything there was to know about self-control. Yet she was now sitting in my office because her old enemy—fear—had her in its grip.

Her terror today dated from the moment when, a few weeks earlier, she had received a diagnosis of kidney cancer. As I explored her past, she told me that her father had raped her on several occasions when she was still a child. The helplessness she now felt confronting her disease was probably in part an echo of what she experienced as a child, when she had no means of escaping a horrific plight.

She had never forgotten the day when she was 6 and she had torn the inside of her thigh on a fence. Her father had taken her to the doctor's office and sat by while she had stitches put in, all the way up to her pubis, without anesthesia. Back home, her father had laid her flat on her stomach and, holding her down with his hand on her nape, raped her for the first time.

Lilian had begun by telling me that, in the course of several years of conventional therapy, she had talked at length about incest and her relationship with her father. She didn't think it would be useful to go back over these old memories. "I'm really over that," she said.

But the connection between that childhood scene—combining the themes of illness, total impotence, and fear—and the anxiety she was now experiencing over her cancer seemed, to me, too powerful to set aside. She finally concurred and agreed to evoke these memories again, using EMDR.

With the first sequence of eye movements, her whole body expressed her childhood terror anew. An idea flashed through her mind: "Wasn't it my fault? Didn't it all start with my fall in the backyard and the fact that my father saw my genitals at the doctor's?" Like most victims of sexual abuse, Lilian felt partly responsible for those dreadful acts. I simply asked her to continue thinking about what she had said and to go through another series of eye movements for 30 seconds. After that sequence, she said she now saw that it was not her fault. She had been only a small child, and her father's role had been to take care of her and protect her. That fact was now perfectly clear. In no way was she responsible for the aggression. She had simply fallen down while playing. What could be more ordinary for an active, adventuresome little girl? Before my very eyes, the adult point of view was beginning to link up with the old distortion that had been preserved in Lilian's emotional brain.

During the next short sequence of eye movements, her emotion changed. Fear gave way to righteous anger. "How could he have done such a thing to me? How could my mother have let him carry on like this for years?" Her body's sensations, which seemed to express as much as her spoken words, also changed. The pressure on the nape of her neck and the fear in the pit of her stomach that she had felt a few minutes earlier now gave way to powerful tensions in her chest and jaw, common by-products of anger.

Several schools of psychotherapy hold that the goal of treatment with rape victims is just that: to lead them to a successful transformation of fear and impotence into legitimate anger at the perpetrator. With EMDR, however, the treatment simply carries on in the same fashion as long as the patient is experiencing inner changes. And indeed, after a few more sequences of eye movements, Lilian saw herself as a little girl who had been emotionally forsaken and sexually abused. She felt deep sorrow and great compassion for that poor little girl. As if she were following the stages of mourning described by Elisabeth Kübler-Ross, her anger changed into sadness.[1] Then she realized that the competent adult she had become could take care of that child. She thought of the ferocity with which she had protected her own children—"like a lionness," she said. Finally, little by little, she told her father's story. During World War II in Holland, while still very young and active in the Resistance, he had been arrested and tortured. Throughout her own childhood, she had heard her mother and her grandparents say that afterwards he had never been the same. Lilian felt a wave of pity and compassion for him welling up in her— even more, of understanding. She now saw him as a man who had had a great thirst for love and compassion that his tough, emotionally hardened wife, much like his parents, had withheld. They had all been trapped in a cultural tradition that left no room for emotions.

A few minutes later, Lilian saw her father as a lost soul, a man who had lived through such harsh realities that "they were enough to drive him crazy." Finally, she saw him as "an old man who can barely walk now. He has such a hard life. I feel sad for him."

Over a bit more than an hour, Lilian's terror as a tiny rape victim had changed to acceptance and even compassion for her aggressor— the most adult perspective conceivable. In that short time, she had moved through all the well-known stages of grief work.

Watching this progression, it seemed as if months or even years of psychotherapy had been condensed into a single 90-minute session.

The stimulation of the adaptive information-processing system seemed to have helped her establish all the necessary connections between past events—those she had lived through as a child—and her perspective as an adult woman. Once she had made those connections, the dysfunctionally stored information was digested—or "metabolized," as biologists say. The memory had lost its power to set off inappropriate emotions. Lilian had even been able to revisit the memory of the first rape and then examine it unflinchingly. "It's as if I'm now simply an observer," she said. " I'm looking at it from afar. It's just a memory, just an image."

Deprived of its dysfunctional "limbic" charge, the memory loses its potency. Its power fades. That, in itself, is a major step forward. Yet, the resolution of old traumas—which we carry around like partially healed wounds—does not end when painful memories are neutralized.

Once she had fully grieved the old pain, Lilian discovered an inner strength that up until then was unsuspected and untapped. She confronted her disease and her grim prognosis with much greater serenity. She became a full-fledged partner with her doctors, and she was able to explore a number of complementary cancer treatments and draw on them with discernment and intelligence. Even more importantly, she was able to go on living a full life throughout her illness. Her psychotherapist, whom she continued to see once a month, was so surprised by Lilian's sudden transformation that she called me one day to find out what had happened. What had we done that was different, in light of the fact that her history of incest had, in theory, been laid to rest earlier, thanks to Lilian's therapy? Results like this don't lie; like most practitioners who've had a similar experience with a patient, Lilian's therapist soon trained in EMDR. Since then, it has become a systematic part of her therapeutic approach.

Three years after these few sessions, Lilian is as alive as ever—perhaps more so—despite surgery, chemotherapy, and radiotherapy.

Thanks to her experience of illness and of her inner strength, she even projects a certain radiance. She has started acting again and has gone back to teaching. And she looks forward to carrying on like this for a long time to come.*

The Children of Kosovo

The adaptive information-processing system works even faster with children. One possible explanation is that their simpler cognitive structures and more limited channels of association accelerate its course.

A few months after the end of the war in Kosovo, I was in Peja acting as a consultant on emotional trauma. One day, I was asked to examine two young adolescents, a brother and sister. During the war, militia had surrounded their house and murdered their father right in front of their eyes. The girl, 15 at the time, had been raped while a revolver was held to her head. Since that horrific event, she had not been able to set foot back in her bedroom. To escape the militia, the boy had fled with his uncle to the roof, where a grenade was thrown up at them, killing his uncle and severely wounding the boy in the abdomen. The militia had left him for dead.

Ever since, the two children had been living in a state of constant anxiety. Even though the war was clearly over and the militia disbanded, the two were sleeping badly, eating little, and refusing to leave the house. The pediatrician who had visited them several times was very concerned about them—all the more so as he was a friend of the family. He didn't know how to help them.

One aspect of my work consisted of teaching doctors how to diagnose PTSD (posttraumatic stress disorder). After one of my lectures,

---

*Obviously, EMDR does not cure cancer. Nevertheless, I know that it played an important role in Lilian's overall treatment, as it has with other patients who were facing a serious and life-threatening illness.

the pediatrician approached me to ask if I would do something for these children. As I listened to the doctor tell me their story, I wondered if there really was anything I could do to help, especially in a foreign language, working through an interpreter. When the children revived these memories themselves, their emotions were intense. Yet, during the initial session, I was surprised to see that immediately after the first series of eye movements, neither of them seemed to be upset any longer. I recall thinking that either their shyness in the presence of the interpreter was blocking their associations, or the trauma had been so great that they could not remain connected with their emotions (in psychiatry, this is referred to as a "dissociation" phenomenon). I was very surprised to hear them say, at the end of the first session, that they could now evoke the images of the aggression without feeling any distress. While obviously a positive sign, this level of "cure" seemed impossible to me. I was certain that within a few days, we would see evidence that nothing had truly been resolved.

A week later, I returned, intending to go on with the treatment and try again, possibly using other scenes as the point of departure. I was astonished when their aunt told me that the very night after our first session, the two children had dined normally for the first time since the incident. Then, they had slept through the night, also for the first time in several months. The girl had even slept in her own room.

I could hardly believe it. I tried to reason it away—the children were probably too polite and docile to tell me that I hadn't done them any good. Or perhaps they simply didn't want to answer any more questions about that painful episode. Perhaps, I thought, the children believed that if they assured me that their symptoms had vanished, they might convince me to leave them alone.

As soon as I saw them, however, I could tell that something truly had changed. They were smiling. They were even laughing, like carefree children of a much simpler place, whereas earlier they had been downcast and sad. They also looked rested. My interpreter, who was a medical student in Belgrade before the war, was convinced that they had undergone a transformation.

Nevertheless, I remained skeptical about the genuine effectiveness of these sessions. Then, a few months later, I met several therapists who specialized in treating PTSD in children. They confirmed to me that children who undergo treatment usually react much faster and show a lot less emotion than adults. In fact, since my experience in Kosovo, one of the first controlled experiments of PTSD treatment in elementary schoolchildren has shown that EMDR is effective in that age group.[2] Even if the results were not as spectacular as those I had witnessed in Kosovo, in this study, EMDR had remarkable effects in children who had not done well with any other approach.

The Battle over EMDR

One of the most curious aspects of the history of the development of EMDR is the resistance it has encountered from academic psychiatry and psychology. In 2000, the most frequently used database for PTSD—the PILOTS' Database at Dartmouth Veterans Adminstration (VA) Hospital—recorded more controlled clinical experiments using EMDR than any other treatment for PTSD. The results of these studies were so impressive that three "meta-analyses"— studies reviewing all the previously published studies—concluded that EMDR was at least as effective as the best existing treatments. In many instances, EMDR also seemed the best tolerated and the fastest method.[3]

Yet, today, EMDR continues to be described as a "controversial" approach in many American university circles (although it is less so in France, Holland, Germany, and England). In the United States, EMDR has even come under attack from some academics as a "fad" and "a marketing technique."[4] In the history of medicine, such controversy is commonplace. When major breakthroughs occur before their theoretical underpinnings can be explained, they systematically encounter violent resistance from entrenched institutions—especially when the treatment is described as "natural" and seems "too simple."

One of the most famous examples of this, which is probably also the most similar to EMDR, is the story of Dr. Philippe Semmelweis. Semmelweis was a Hungarian physician, who showed the importance of sterile techniques (asepsis) in childbirth, 20 years before Lister and Pasteur discovered the concept of germs. At that time, in the maternity clinic where the young Dr. Semmelweis was an assistant professor, more than one woman in three died of puerperal fever in the days after giving birth. The poorest women in Vienna, the only ones to have recourse to such clinics, went there only under duress, because they knew all too well the risks they were taking.

Dr. Semmelweis had the extraordinary insight to suggest the following experiment: All the doctors, who often carried out dissection with bare hands just before attending a birth, had to wash their hands with lime before touching their patients' genital area. He had a great deal of difficulty imposing that idea. Because these events took place before the discovery of germs, there was no logical reason to believe that apparently clean hands could transmit something invisible and odorless that could cause death.

In any case, the results of his experiment were extraordinary. In a month, mortality dropped from one patient in three to one in twenty. But the principal outcome of the experiment for Dr. Semmelweis was his dismissal. His colleagues, who found it tedious to clean their hands with lime, rebelled and got him fired. As there was no plausible explanation for such results at the time, Dr. Semmelweis and his improbable idea were mocked, despite his brilliant demonstration. He died on the verge of insanity, only a few years before the discoveries that finally enabled Pasteur and Lister to

provide a scientific explanation for what Dr. Semmelweis had discovered empirically.

More recently, in psychiatry, it took more than 20 years for the
FDA (Food and Drug Administration) to recognize the benefits of
lithium for the treatment of bipolar disorder (also referred to as
"manic-depressive syndrome"). Lithium was simply a "natural mineral
salt" without known benefits for the central nervous system, and its
mechanism was not understood. Thus, lithium's use as a therapy encountered stiff resistance from conventional medicine.*

In an even more recent example, at the beginning of the 1980s,
the discovery that stomach ulcers might be caused by a bacterium—
H. pylori—and treated with antibiotics was held up to ridicule at medical conventions. Despite compelling results, it took more than 10
years for this new idea to be accepted.†

EMDR and Dream Sleep

The fact is, we still do not understand how EMDR produces these impressive results. Robert Stickgold, M.D., Ph.D., from the Harvard
Laboratory of Neurophysiology, has put forward the hypothesis that
eye movements and other forms of stimulation that elicit a similar
physiological response (the reorienting of attention) play a major role
in reorganizing memory in the brain. This response may take place
just as often during sleep—and dreaming—as in the course of an

---

*An Australian, John F. J. Cade, M.D., had demonstrated the effects of lithium in bipolar disorder
in 1949. But American psychiatrists began to use it only in the mid-1960s, and it was officially ap-
proved by the FDA only in 1974. As of 2004, the mechanism of action of lithium remains relatively
mysterious, although several promising leads have recently opened up with the discovery of its effects on genetic transcription and inhibition of protein-kinase C. (Manji, H. K., W. Z. Potter, et
al. (1995), "Signal transduction pathways: molecular targets for lithium's actions," *Archives of General
Psychiatry*, no. 52, pp. 531–543)

†Another Australian, Barry Marshall, M.D., made this discovery. Exasperated by his colleagues' refusal to believe his observations, he ended up swallowing a test tube of concentrated bacteria to
prove that it would provoke an ulcer, which it did.

EMDR session. In an article about sleep physiology in the journal *Science*, Dr. Stickgold and his colleagues have suggested that such forms of stimulation activate the associations linking up memories that are interconnected through emotions.[5] Dr. Stickgold thinks that similar mechanisms may be brought into play by the sensory stimulation generated through EMDR.[6] Other researchers have shown that, from their outset, eye movements also induce a response of "forced relaxation," leading to an immediate drop in heart rate and a rise in body temperature.[7] This suggests that EMDR stimulation—like the practice of cardiac coherence—reinforces the activity of the parasympathetic nervous system.

Dr. Stickgold's theory possibly also explains why EMDR may work when using techniques other than eye movements for stimulating attention. In addition to the eyes, the auditory system is also stimulated during dream sleep, and involuntary muscular contractions on the surface of the skin also occur.[8] In fact, instead of eye movements, some clinicians use sounds alternating left to right through headphones. Or they stimulate the skin by tapping or applying vibrations alternatively to the right and left hand. Indeed, as we will see in chapter 8, stimulation through the skin has been found to directly alter activity in the emotional brain.

My own conviction is that eye movements—or other forms of stimulation that capture attention—help patients stay focused on the present while reexperiencing emotions that belong to the past. It may be this dual state of attention—one foot in the past and one foot in the present—that triggers a reorganization of the traumatic memory in the brain.[9]

Clearly, there is still much to learn about the adaptive information-processing system and different ways to help it perform or accelerate its work of digestion. In the meantime, EMDR is rapidly gaining ground, thanks to the growing number of scientific studies demonstrating its effectiveness. Today, EMDR is officially recognized as an effective treatment by the American Psychological Association,[10] by the International Society for Traumatic Stress Studies (ISTSS—which selects recommended treatments for PTSD on the basis of established scientific criteria),[11] by the Department of Health in the United Kingdom,[12] and by the Departments of Health in Israel and Northern Ireland in their reports on effective psychological interventions after attacks.[13, 14] In France, Sweden, Germany, and Holland, medical schools and departments of psychology are starting to teach EMDR.

Treatment with EMDR is often usefully combined with other forms of therapy, such as cognitive-behavior therapy, marital therapy (to help one of the partners to get through an old trauma that poisons the relationship), and psychodynamic or psychoanalytic therapy. Certainly, no conflict exists between EMDR and these other approaches to therapy. Quite the contrary: By bringing in the body and its own memories and conflicts, EMDR is a useful and complementary tool to make progress more quickly and easily.*

Of course, among the large number of studies looking at the effects of EMDR, some have had negative results. Some have even found no difference between EMDR sessions done with and without eye movements. The difficulty in measuring the exact effect of a treatment and understanding its exact mechanisms is a reality that is shared by all of medicine. This gap in knowledge between what works and how it works is certainly true of antidepressants as well: Several studies have suggested that, on the basis of the data made available to the FDA, antidepressants are barely better than placebos, yet most of us who use antidepressants find them to be useful under the appropriate circumstances.[15] In coming years, it will be important to continue weighing any new evidence about this fascinating new approach to healing emotional pain.

---

*As a testimonial to this natural symbiosis, in June 2002, Francine Shapiro, Ph.D., received the Sigmund Freud Prize—one of the most prestigious distinctions that a psychotherapist can obtain—awarded jointly by the World Psychotherapy Council and the City of Vienna.

"Small-t" Traumas Leave a Lasting Trace

In the meantime, the discovery of an effective way to heal trauma may change the practice of psychiatry and psychotherapy. At the end of the 19th century, Pierre Janet, a leading figure of European psychiatry, and then Sigmund Freud both arrived at a daring hypothesis: A major share of the psychological disturbance encountered every day in clinical practice—depression, anxiety, eating disorders, alcoholism, and drug abuse—originated in traumatic events. This theory was a major contribution, but unfortunately, it was not followed by a method of treatment that could quickly relieve the victims of emotional trauma.

Now, when EMDR eliminates the dysfunctional trace of emotions, the symptoms of psychological disturbance often vanish completely and a new personality can emerge. With an intervention that can treat the cause of symptoms rather than simply help manage them, the whole approach to patients can be transformed—all the more so because traumas "with a small 't' " are very common and they are the cause of many other symptoms besides PTSD.

A study carried out in an emergency department in Australia illustrates the manifold effects of "minor" emotional shocks. For a year, researchers followed up the victims of automobile accidents treated in the department. At the end of the year, these patients underwent a series of psychological examinations. More than half of them had developed psychiatric disorders since their accident. Of all the disorders noted, PTSD was the *least* common. These people were suffering most often from simple depression, ordinary anxiety attacks, or phobias. A good number had even developed pure eating disorders, or alcohol or drug abuse, without other conditions.[16] The major lesson of this study is that PTSD is not the only disorder—far from it—requiring an examination of past events that may have left emotional scars with enduring pain. All forms of depression or anxiety call for a systematic effort to search out the cause of today's symptoms in the patient's past history. Only then can the greatest possible number of these unresolved emotional traces be eliminated.

Vera, the nurse whose story I told in the preceding chapter, was so worried about her physical appearance that she thought only a general liposuction would allow her to look at herself in a mirror. We started the first series of eye movements precisely on that image of herself, naked, in the mirror. She had rated it as "unbearable," with a distress level of 10/10. (She actually said, "15!" out of 10.)

We did the first sequence of eye movements as she focused on that disturbing image. The first thing that came to her mind was the memory of her ex-husband referring to her pregnancy-related weight gain with disgust. She heard his words again: "You're the ugliest thing I've ever seen. . . ." As that recollection returned, the tears she had held back for 3 years poured out of her. We simply continued with another sequence of eye movements that lasted 2 minutes or so. Then an expression of anger came over her face. She turned to me and looked a bit disconcerted: "How could he have said something like that when it was a little person inside of me, and it was his child?" Rather than allow her to speak too much, I asked her to simply think about that and to begin the eye movements again.

After a few minutes, she started to smile. I asked her what she was thinking. "That he's still a useless piece of crap! I can't stand him!" she laughingly exclaimed. She did a few more series of eye movements, and I led her back to the initial image of her nude body in the mirror. I asked her what she saw now. Breathing normally, in a calm voice, she said, "The body of a normal 30-year-old woman who has had two children." Her entire being seemed to be at peace.

Despite these dramatic results, we cannot look at EMDR as a panacea. In my experience, this technique does not work as well when symptoms do not have their roots in painful past events. In such cases, EMDR can still be useful, but the results are neither as rapid nor as impressive.*

On the other hand, other natural methods also have a direct impact on the body's biological rhythms. Indeed, the emotional brain is not only subject to heart variations and to the influence of sleep and dreams. The emotional brain is part of a larger whole whose rhythms it also shares: the rhythm of the sun, alternating night and day; the monthly periodicity of the moon, influencing the menstrual cycle; and the longer rhythms of the seasons. As we will now see, these longer cycles also offer a pathway to emotional well-being.

---

*EMDR is not indicated for severe depressions clearly of biological origin; for psychoses, such as schizophrenia or others; or for dementia.

7

The Energy of Light:
Resetting Your Biological Clock

Dr. Frederick Cook was a seasoned explorer of the great North in the 19th century. When his ship and his crew became stuck in the Arctic, he never lost hope about surviving in a harsh physical environment. However, Dr. Cook did not expect the emotional challenge awaiting him and his men.

Stuck at the beginning of winter, they were facing 68 days of consecutive darkness. In his journal, Dr. Cook noted: "The days are growing rapidly shorter and the nights only too noticeably longer. . . . It is the discouraging veil of blackness, falling over the sparkling whiteness of earlier nights, which sends a vein of despair running through our souls." He found his men becoming gradually more and more apathetic and pessimistic as the winter nights deepened. Dr. Cook eventually resorted to direct exposure to an open fire as his primary method of treatment for the spirits of the crew, and he noted that this benefited them perhaps more because of the light it offered than because of the heat.

Conversely, Dr. Cook also observed the liberating influence of longer days, with the arrival of spring, upon the instinctual life of the Eskimos: "The passions of these people are periodical, and their courtship is usually carried on soon after the return of the sun; in fact, at this time, they almost tremble from the intensity of their passions and for several weeks, most of their time is taken up in gratifying them."[1]

The impact of light and sun on mood and human drives was recorded well before Dr. Cook, even during biblical times. That we seem happier in the spring than in the ebb of winter is such an obvious fact that we forget that it has deep implications about how to improve our mood and enhance our energy level. Light directly influences, even controls, essential functions of the emotional brain. For animals living in the wild, the length of night and day controls when they sleep and when they rise. It also controls most vital drives, including appetite for food and sex, as well as their appetite for exploration and novelty.

Experiments in the laboratory easily show that light is *the* essential controlling factor, as opposed to changes in ambient temperature, or exposure to pollens, or other factors related to the changing of seasons. Light penetrates the brain through the eyes, and the neural impulse is transmitted to a special group of cells in the hypothalamus, one of the main output nuclei of the emotional brain. As the hormone control center of the body, the hypothalamus directly influences appetite, sex drive, sleep cycles, menstrual cycles, body heat regulation, and mood.

Because we share our limbic structures with animals, exposure to light influences our drives and our biological functions in a similar way. Of course, artificial light has freed us from the strict cycles of sleeping and waking imposed by the appearance and disappearance of the sun. However, even on a typical overcast day, outdoor daylight is 5 to 20 times more bright than the light from indoor fixtures. Because of this, artificial light cannot replace the entrainment that the sun exerts on our biological rhythms.

All the Rhythms of the Body

Sleepiness, dreaming, body temperature, hormone secretion, and digestion are all regulated according to a 24-hour cycle that is largely independent of when we actually sleep. This constant 24-hour cycle is the reason we experience jet lag when we cross time zones. Even though we may still sleep from 11 P.M. to 7 A.M. in the new time zone, the sleeping period of the first few nights does not correspond to the period of the dreaming cycle, the body temperature cycle, or the cortisol-release cycle, which have all continued to follow their own "clock." The same thing happens when we go to bed 4 hours later than usual after a party on a Saturday night. We may still have slept 8 hours, but the period of sleep was "out of sync" with the other underlying cycles of the body. The last 4 hours of sleep, for example, took place while our cortisol level and body temperature had already started to rise. This is why we feel ragged and worn down the next day (well, that and the wine, of course).

However, most of these internal cycles can be directly trained by exposure to light. Just as sunflowers turn to the sun every day, our hypothalamus is designed to orient itself to the changing rhythm of shortening and lengthening days of seasons. When oriented properly, the hypothalamus's control over the secretion of hormones and neuropeptides can be very precise.*

When days grow shorter in winter, about one person in three notices changes in certain basic drives that are controlled by the

---

*The secretion of melatonin at night, for example, starts within minutes after dark and continues until any light signal is registered. Once light is recognized, the melatonin flow stops within seconds. (Moore, R. Y. (1996). "Neural control of the pineal gland," *Behavioural Brain Research* 73(1–2): 125–130)

hypothalamus. The changes look a bit like symptoms of hibernation: craving for carbohydrates (bread, pasta, potatoes, sweets),
longer sleep, decreased energy, decreased sex drive, low motivation
to take on new projects, and sluggish thought processes. For 10 percent of the population living above 40 degrees of latitude (New
York City in North America, Madrid in Europe), these symptoms
take on the proportion of a clinical depression between November
and March.[2] The symptoms of this "seasonal affective disorder" are
strikingly more *physical* than psychological, since they reflect
changes in physiological drives more than consequences of emotional pain.

When Frank came to see me, I was struck by the apparent lack of
psychological explanation for the symptoms that had plagued him
for the last 2 years. A successful businessman in his forties, Frank
was handsome and friendly, clearly comfortable talking about himself, and at ease with the very private questions I was asking about his
personal history. He had suffered from the usual ups and downs of
life, but I could not find any lingering pain from these past painful
events. His business had been stressful at times, but it had all remained within bounds that were familiar to him, a level of difficulty
he had often experienced as "challenging and stimulating" rather than
overwhelming.

Yet, for the past 2 years, Frank had consulted multiple physicians
to get relief from a progressive and debilitating bout of chronic fatigue, clouded thinking, fretful sleep, and pain in his neck and shoul-
ders. These symptoms had eventually led him to work only part time.
Because he had the classic "trigger points" along his back and neck
(areas the size of a dime that are exquisitely sensitive to pressure by
the examining doctor), Frank had been diagnosed with "fibromyalgia."

Fibromyalgia is a poorly understood condition that associates several features of depression with disabling fatigue and pain. The condition is dreaded by patients and physicians alike because it tends to

be chronic in nature and to respond only partially to a variety of conventional treatments, including antidepressants. Patients who suffer from fibromyalgia experience themselves as *physically* sick and resent the pressure from physicians to see a psychiatrist or to take antidepressants.

I didn't feel much more equipped to help Frank than my many colleagues, conventional and alternative, who had already showered him with multiple different suggestions. Under various physicians' treatment, he'd tried everything from nutrition to psychotherapy to anti-inflammatory drugs, but nothing had been of much help. As I listened to his story, I was struck by one detail in his recollection of how his condition had started. He clearly remembered that his problems started after a bout of unsatisfying sleep, and he had continued to develop particular trouble with getting up in the morning. This situation had preceded his problems with pain. Furthermore, the sleep issue had started in early December, when daylight is shortening rapidly.

Just as my other colleagues had done, I suggested to Frank that he try yet another treatment method. I told him that perhaps this one might just help, and that it certainly couldn't possibly hurt him, not even inconvenience him. This was my first experience with using artificial simulation of dawn as a treatment, and I never expected it would be so helpful.

Since the late 1980s, researchers at the National Institute of Mental Health and elsewhere have experimented with light therapy for depressive syndromes that have a clear-cut seasonal pattern. They have demonstrated that 30 minutes of daily exposure to a bright light device (10,000 lux, or roughly 20 times the brightness of a regular lightbulb) can reverse the symptoms of seasonal depression within 2 weeks. However, patients often complain about having to stay in front of a light box for 30 minutes every day, and long-term compliance with this treatment is fairly disappointing. In the last 10 years, David Avery, M.D., at the University of Washington in Seattle, has pioneered the research of a new approach to light therapy. Instead of a brutal exposure to 10,000 lux immediately upon waking up, it may be possible to let the soft onset of a simulated dawn take care of awakening the brain.

Dawn Simulation

It's 6 A.M., and your room is in total darkness. Suddenly, a screeching alarm clock tears through the silence and propels you out of a dream. With heavy eyelids, you throw your hand at the alarm clock, trying to quiet that unwelcome intrusion. "Five more minutes," you plead wearily. The day isn't starting very well. But is there any alternative?

Yes, you do have another choice: a dawn simulation device. Need to wake up at 6 A.M.? Beginning at 5:15, the device starts to slowly light up your room. Softly, progressively, it simulates the appearance—slow at first, then faster and faster—of a natural sunrise, the signal to which your emotional brain has been wired to awaken during millions of years of evolution on Earth. After several hours of night, your eyes have become so sensitive to light signals that they can detect this smooth transition even from behind closed eyelids. When the first rays of light begin to appear, they register with the hypothalamus and begin to prepare our brain for a soft transition into awakening. Dreams begin to wrap up, body temperature and cortisol begin to rise, and, as the light intensity reaches higher levels, the pattern of typical electrical activity of neurons during sleep progressively transitions into that of light awakening and then of complete arousal.

Recent studies in people who suffer from winter depression suggest that dawn simulation may be even *more* effective than morning exposure to a high-intensity light box.[3] Perhaps it is because dawn simulation harnesses the natural regulation mechanisms of the body's circadian rhythms, as opposed to jerking them with abrupt exposure to artificial light after awakening in complete darkness. For those who are afraid of so much softness, some devices are equipped with a "backup alarm" that rings at the end of the dawn period. (See chapter 15 for more information on purchasing dawn simulators.)

With great anticipation, Frank tried his dawn simulator. He plugged his usual bedside lamp into the small electronic device that can be set like an alarm clock. The following morning, he found himself awakened by the bright light of his lamp before his regular alarm clock went off. Within a week, he noticed a different pattern to his awakenings. He would typically still be dreaming when he'd find himself coming out of the dream, though barely so, realizing that it was morning, and then slipping back into the dream again. This dipping in and out of consciousness would happen once or twice before he'd notice his body and his mind were more and more awake and less and less interested in going back to sleep.

Within 2 weeks, Frank found himself more alert during the day and able to think more clearly. His mood was picking up. After a few months, his new wake-up technique even started to help with his pain, though that never completely disappeared. Frank described his experience in a note to the company that manufactures his dawn simulator: "I can't begin to tell you what difference this light has made in my life. I have found no other approach that has helped me as much. The fact that it is completely natural is an extra bonus, as I do not tolerate medications well. . . . I don't understand how it works, but I certainly feel more rested, coherent, and energized when I awaken, and that makes all the difference in my day, every day."[4]

Perhaps the most fascinating aspect of dawn simulation is how important it may be to all of us, depressed or not, stressed or not. As a medical student, my first exposure to psychiatry was at the Stanford Medical Center, where I learned about sleep, its different phases, and its relation to mental problems. Our teacher, Vincent Zarcone, M.D., was one of the leading sleep researchers in the world. He described to us how dream sleep—also referred to as REM (rapid eye movement) sleep or "paradoxical sleep" because the brain looks fully awake even though the body is maximally relaxed—takes place mostly during the later part of the night, as the brain and body are preparing to awaken. This is the reason why we often wake up from a dream in the morning.

I thought about this for a while. I had noticed for a long time how unpleasant it felt to be awakened from a dream by an alarm clock in the morning and how much better it was to wake up *after* the dream had completed its natural course. After the lecture, I asked Dr. Zarcone if anyone had ever invented a device that would prevent the alarm clock from ringing while people are still dreaming. With all the physiology that we now understood about REM sleep, it seemed it must be possible to detect if someone was still in this phase of sleep and to simply delay the ringing of the clock until the dream ended. Dr. Zarcone laughed and his eyes had the sparkle of someone who recognized exactly why I was asking, as if he had wondered about this many times for himself, too. "That would be nice, wouldn't it?" he said. "But I don't know of any such device and I think anything you'd come up with would be much too cumbersome for everyday use." This was 20 years ago. Today, dawn simulators seem like such an obvious answer to this problem that it makes one wonder why nobody came up with the idea earlier. Why should anyone wake up to the abrupt screeching of an alarm clock that jerks all of our biological rhythms out of their natural flow when these devices can make us land delicately on the shoreline of the day, according to the laws of millions of years of evolution?

Just as intriguing is the possibility that adding this seamless technology to our way of living could bring benefits that reach beyond seasonal changes in mood or softer mornings. Traditional light therapy can be helpful in a variety of conditions. In some studies, it has been found to stabilize menstrual cycles, to improve the quality of sleep, to reduce the carbohydrate craving and the frequency of binges that some experience during the winter, and to enhance the response to antidepressants in people who are otherwise resistant to treatment.[5] Recently, researchers at the University of California, San Diego, have found that just 5 days of early morning bright light exposure could increase testosterone secretion in healthy men by more than 60 percent.[6]

None of these effects have been studied yet with dawn simulation, only with the usual exposure to a bright light box. If such results were replicated with dawn simulation, they would suggest that we could all significantly improve our well-being simply by changing the way we wake up in the morning. No doubt this will be an active area of research in the coming years.

If light can entrain our body's rhythms through its control over the emotional brain, 5,000 years of traditional Chinese and Tibetan medicine suggest yet another powerful way to modulate the flow of energy between the mind and the body. In spite of its ultimate simplicity and elegance, this system of medicine is just starting to be explored by Western science. And we are already learning quite a bit about its mysterious efficacy.

8

The Power of Qi: Acupuncture Directly Affects the Emotional Brain

Like two people who are meant to be friends but who do not realize it the first time they meet, during my first encounter with acupuncture, I missed my chance.

I was still a medical student in Paris in the early 1980s, before I went to the United States to continue my training. One of my professors at the time was just back from China. He had read a book by the Frenchman Soulié de Morant—among the first to introduce acupuncture to the West[1]—and had decided to find out about it for himself. To document his findings, he had shot a Super 8 film of an operation in a Beijing hospital.

With 200 fellow students, I watched, agape, as a woman talked quietly with a surgeon who was removing a cyst the size of a melon from her open abdomen. The only anesthesia consisted of a few very fine needles inserted under her skin. Obviously, we had never seen anything like it. Yet, as soon as the film was over and the light was back on, we all quickly forgot what we had just seen. Maybe it was possible in China, but here? . . . It was too remote from what we knew and from the vast stores of Western medical knowledge remaining for us to acquire. Too remote and too esoteric. I did not give that film another thought for 15 years, until the day when I went to India, to Dharamsala, the seat of the Government of Tibet in Exile, in the foothills of the Himalaya.

I visited the Institute of Tibetan Medicine and talked with a practitioner about his views on depression and anxiety. "You Westerners," he said, "have a vision of emotional problems that's all topsy-turvy. You're always surprised to see that what you call depression or anxiety or stress has physical symptoms. You talk about fatigue, weight gain or loss, irregular heartbeats, as if they were physical manifestations of an emotional problem. To us, the opposite is true. Sadness, loss of self-esteem, guilt feelings, the absence of pleasure, can be mental manifestations of a physical problem."

True, I had never thought about it this way. And his view of depression was just as plausible as the Western one. He went on: "In truth, both of these views are wrong. To us, emotional symptoms *and* physical ones are simply two sides of the same thing: an imbalance in the circulation of energy, the Qi."

At that point, he lost me. Grounded by my training in the Cartesian tradition, which marks a strict distinction between the "mental" and the "physical," I was not yet ready to talk about "Qi" (pronounced "chi"). Nor was I ready to imagine an underlying, governing "energy" affecting both the physical and the mental realm—especially one that could not be measured with objective instruments. But my Tibetan colleague went on: "There are three ways to influence Qi: through meditation—which regenerates it; through nutrition and medicinal herbs; and, directly, with acupuncture. We often treat what you call depression with acupuncture. It works very well provided that patients follow the treatment long enough."

But I was not listening to him anymore. He was talking to me about meditation, herbs, and needles. We were no longer on the same wavelength. Besides, as soon as he referred to the length of treatment, I immediately imagined that it must involve the placebo effect, responses patients have to treatments that do not contain any active agent. Placebos generally work well when patients are being taken care of regularly and kindly, and with convincing displays of technical competence. Since this is exactly what an acupuncturist does, it seemed obvious to me that any response to acupuncture must be a placebo effect. Once I had reached this conclusion, I just listened to him politely and then found an excuse to move on with my day. That was the second chance I missed—but this one had left a trace in my memory.

The third encounter took place in Pittsburgh a year or two afterwards. One Saturday afternoon in the street, I met a patient I had seen only once, in the outpatient clinic of the hospital. She had been suffering from quite a serious depression, but she had refused to take the antidepressants I offered her. We'd gotten along well, nevertheless, so when I saw her, I asked her how she was now, if she was feeling any better. She looked at me smiling, but a bit unsure as to whether she could be frank with me or not. I must've seemed open, because she finally told me that she had decided to see an acupuncturist. She said she'd had a few sessions over 4 weeks, and now she was fine.

If I had not had that conversation with the Tibetan doctor in Dharamsala, I surely would have attributed her "cure" to the placebo effect. As I already mentioned, in depression, the placebo effect is common—so common, in fact, that it takes about three clinical studies comparing an antidepressant to a placebo for one of them to show that the medication is superior.[2] But the conversation in Dharamsala came back to me immediately and I was a bit annoyed, I must admit, that a treatment different from mine had been more useful. I decided to find out more about this strange practice. What I learned about the extent of its impact on the nature of body and mind still staggers me.

Science and Needles

First of all, with 5,000 years of documented practice, acupuncture is probably the oldest medical technique in use on our planet. Over the past 50 centuries, a great many placebos have come to light—ineffective plants (some of them toxic), snake oils, tortoise shell powders, and so on. But none, to my knowledge, has survived everyday medical practice for so long. When I started to take acupuncture seriously, I discovered that in 1978, the World Health Organization had published a report officially recognizing acupuncture as an acceptable, effective medical practice. Moreover, a report from the National Institutes of Health circulating in academic circles at the time concluded that acupuncture was effective for at least certain disorders, such as postoperative pain, and nausea during pregnancy or chemotherapy. Since then, a report from the British Medical Association, published in 2000, has come to similar conclusions, while lengthening the list of indications to include, for example, backache.[3]

Then I discovered that, if acupuncture really was a placebo, rabbits were just as sensitive to it as human beings. Several experiments have clearly demonstrated that a rabbit can be "anesthetized" by stimulating points on its paw corresponding to those that block pain in human beings. Still more convincing: When cerebrospinal fluid (the fluid that bathes the brain and the spinal cord) of an "anesthetized" rabbit is injected into a second rabbit, the second animal no longer feels pain either. (And this is not true of an injection of placebo fluid.) It is thus proven that, at the very least, acupuncture induces the secretion of substances by the brain that can block the experience of pain, beyond any placebo effect.[4]

The international scientific literature also contained a whole range of research studies confirming the efficacy of acupuncture for a variety of problems. These not only included depression, anxiety, and insomnia, but also intestinal disorders, tobacco and heroin addiction, and even infertility in women (doubling, for example, the success rate of artificial insemination). There was even a study in the *Journal of the American Medical Association* showing that a fetus in a breach position can be turned around in its mother's uterus, in 80 percent of cases, with the stimulation of a single acupuncture point.[5]

A Personal Encounter

In the wake of these compelling findings about acupuncture, even more surprising studies would be undertaken (we will return to them further on), but this information was already enough to inspire me to find out more about acupuncture. I had heard of a rather unusual practitioner, a certain Christine, who treated patients with emotional problems with "five-elements acupuncture." She was the one who had taken care of my patient with depression to such good effect. So I thought it was logical to begin with her.

Christine was not a physician, but she had been practicing acupuncture for 25 years. Her office was a white-walled room in the tower of a country house surrounded by trees. Sunlight poured through the many windows at all hours of the day. Two canvas armchairs sat side by side, near a low table. There was no desk, just a massage table dressed with a Native American cover in tones of red, pink, and purple. On the wall, a message greeted me: "Illness is an adventure. Acupuncture gives you the swords, but the fighting is up to you."

While asking me about my personal history, Christine took notes for an hour. She asked strange questions. For example, she asked me if I tolerated heat better than cold; if I preferred raw or cooked food; if I had more energy in the morning or in the evening. Next she took my pulse at length, on both sides at once, with her eyes shut as if to concentrate better. She even did it several times. After a few minutes, she said, "You know you have a heart murmur, don't you? It's not serious. It's been there for a long time and it doesn't bother you."

Now, hearing a slight heart murmur with a stethoscope is already pretty hard, but I had never met a cardiologist who could detect one by taking the pulse. Under ordinary circumstances, I would have taken that for bluff, but I suddenly recalled a cardiologist colleague I had seen for a completely different problem 15 years earlier who had told me the same thing. He had listened to my heart for a good 5 minutes and then said, "You have a slight heart murmur. Nobody will hear it, in my opinion, but if somebody tells you about it, keep in mind that it doesn't matter." And I had not thought about it since. How had this woman, in her shaman's setting, identified mine simply with her fingers?

Next, she asked me to lie down almost completely undressed on the massage table. I essentially had a morphological type and a "yang" personality, she explained. I didn't have enough "yin" in my kidneys and "too much Qi" in my liver, she also said. As she spoke she used a small cloth moistened with alcohol to wipe different points on my body. She said the stimulation from needles inserted in these points was going to "foster a better balance in my energy and in the relationship among my organs."

The points she had chosen were essentially on my feet and tibias, my hands and wrists—without any clear connection, then, to the liver or the kidneys. Naturally, I was worried about the needles. I was surprised to see that they were almost hair-fine. Anyhow, I did not feel anything when she inserted each one skillfully, with a quick, sharp movement, under my skin. Not even the sensation of a mosquito bite. Nothing. It was only later, when she turned one lightly or pushed down on it, that I felt a slight electric discharge, deeper down. Strangely, Christine sometimes seemed to feel it before I did. She said: "Ah, there we are. I've got it." And in fact, a half a second later, I felt the electricity that seemed to have "found" the needle, like lightning that has homed in on the lightning rod. She called this sensation "Dai Qi," and explained that it was the signal that she had reached the point she was looking for. "What you feel is the Qi in movement, attracted to the needle," she explained.

As she handled a needle on my foot, I felt sudden brief pressure in the lower back. "Yes," she told me, "I'm on the meridian for the kidney. I told you that your kidney needed yin. That's what I'm trying to work on."

I was fascinated by these "meridians"—"virtual" lines running up and down the body that had been described 2,500 years ago. Meridians do not correspond to any material reality in the body, such as the arterial and venous systems, or the lymphatic ducts, or even the dermatomes. Yet they were so clearly manifest in my own body.

A few minutes and 10 needles later on, a sensation of calm and relaxation began to spread throughout my body. The feeling was a little like the well-being that follows intense physical effort. At the end of the session, I had a sense of renewed energy; I was eager to do lots of things, call friends, go out to dinner, . . .

Christine took my pulse again. "The yin in your kidneys has increased as it needed to. I'm pleased," she said, smiling. Then she looked at me. "You need to take more time to relax. You don't take enough care of yourself. It's constant activity that is using it up. Do you meditate? That builds it back up, you know." She also advised me to change my diet and suggested some medicinal herbs—exactly what my Tibetan colleague had done with his patients in Dharamsala.

Acupuncture and the Brain

Although first explored at the Massachusetts General Hospital by the team of Dr. Kathleen Hui, what really sparked scientific interest in acupuncture was the publication of an article by a different group of scientists in *Proceedings of the National Academy of Sciences* a few years later.[6] Only members of the American Academy of Sciences or their "guests" may publish their work in this select journal. Professor Zhang-Hee Cho, Ph.D., at the University of California, Irvine, a researcher in neuroscience and brain imaging, set out to test the 2,500-year-old theory which held that stimulating the little toe with an acupuncture needle improves, of all things, vision. He put 10 healthy people in a scanner and began testing his machine by flashing a black and white checkerboard in front of their eyes. This is the strongest known stimulation of the visual system. Indeed, the images showed major activation of the occipital region, specifically that of the visual cortex, located at the very back of the brain. In all the participants, the flashing checkerboard set off a strong increase in the activity of that region of the brain, which ceased when the stimulation ceased. As expected, their brains' reactions were totally normal.

Then Dr. Cho asked an experienced acupuncturist to stimulate the point known in Chinese medicine textbooks as "Bladder 67," located on the outside edge of the little toe and reputed to improve vision. To the team's surprise, when the needle was handled in the traditional way—twirled quickly between the acupuncturist's fingers—the scanner images showed activity in the same region of the brain, the visual cortex. True, the activity was less intense than with the checkerboards, but it was pronounced enough to pass all statistical tests. Next, Dr. Cho wanted to make sure that this result was not the product of either the researchers' or the subjects' hallucination. So, he then stimulated a point on the big toe that did not correspond to a meridian. And no activation of the visual regions occurred. Convincing, but that was still not the end of the experiment.

One of the most astonishing concepts in traditional Chinese and Tibetan medicine is the idea of different "morphopsychological types," in particular the "yin" and the "yang" types. These two dominant types are identified on the basis of each person's preferences for cold or hot settings, for certain foods, and for certain times of day, and also on the basis of their physical appearance—even on the shape of their calves. Ancient texts state that stimulation of certain acupuncture points can have exactly opposite effects with different patients, depending on their type—hence the importance of identifying them beforehand. Dr. Cho therefore asked the acupuncturist to identify each subject's type, then he observed the effects of stimulating "Bladder 67" on the little toe of both the yin and the yang subjects. Finally, he checked to see if both groups reacted in the same way when they saw the flashing checkerboard: showing activation of the visual cortex, then inactivity when the stimulation stopped. The yin subjects all had the same type of response when their "Bladder 67" was stimulated—activation with stimulation and return to normal when the activation stopped. However—incredible as it seemed— the yang subjects showed the *opposite* effect. Stimulation with the needle "deactivated" the visual cortex, and when the stimulation stopped, the visual cortex returned to normal.

The distinction of yin-yang does not correspond to anything known in modern physiology. It was nevertheless able to predict, as the ancient Chinese texts suggest, that the brain would respond in exactly opposite ways to the same stimulation with the same needle at the same acupuncture point. This outcome is so surprising that most Western scientists prefer, as I chose to do 25 years ago, not to think about it.

To Paul, acupuncture was not a theoretical matter. He had been suffering from depression for years and had been taking a standard antidepressant for months, to no effect. He had come to see Thomas Ost, L.Ac., the acupuncturist at the Center for Complementary Medicine of our hospital, for his backache. Although the primary treatment was for pain, Ost knew about Paul's depression from his intake questions, so he offered to add two points on the skull that several Chinese studies had suggested worked with depression.[7] Halfway through the first session, Paul later declared, he could "feel a layer of fog lifting" that had prevented him from thinking. He felt lighter and a little more confident, even if he still felt the lump in his throat that he always associated with his periods of depression.

After several weekly sessions, he felt the other layers gradually lift as well. Then, in turn, his throat cleared. Little by little, he started to sleep better. His energy came back for the first time in 2 years. Finally, his self-confidence returned, along with his desire to spend time with his wife and daughters and to take on new projects. As in the Chinese studies, his symptoms seemed to respond to acupuncture in the same way and at the same pace as to the antidepressants to which they had been compared.

Naturally, in order to be safe, Paul had never stopped taking the antidepressant his doctor had prescribed, so it is possible that it was his medicine, kicking in late, that produced those changes. However, the fact that the first signs of relief appeared at the first session of acupuncture suggests that the needles were responsible for triggering his recovery. And of course, the two treatments may have been mutually reinforcing: The acupuncture may have stimulated the self-healing mechanisms of the emotional brain while the antidepressants also did their work.

Acupuncturists, both Western and Asian, know very well that their art is particularly useful in the relief of stress, anxiety, and depression. Yet, in the West, these particular uses are the least recognized and the least studied. The rare Western studies are positive. Acupuncture has even been found to control patients' anxiety before an operation, as an alternative to anxiolytic medication (such as Valium or Ativan), which was shown in a study conducted at a Yale University Hospital.[8] But acupuncture's use is still very limited, doubtless because, as with EMDR, we do not understand its mechanisms of action very well.

At Harvard, one such mechanism has just come to light. Kathleen Hui, M.D., with the help of a team from Massachusetts General Hospital (one of the largest centers for functional brain imaging in the world), has demonstrated how acupuncture can directly affect the emotional brain. By stimulating a single point—located on the back of the hand between the thumb and the index finger—she showed the partial anesthesia of the circuits of pain and fear. This point—"Large Intestine 4," called "negu" or "hoku" in ancient Chinese texts—is one of the oldest and most frequently used by all the acupuncturists in the world. It is well-known, in fact, for controlling pain and anxiety. Stimulation through the skin—as happens in EMDR when the skin is used for stimulation rather than eye movements—thus seems able to "speak to" and act on the emotional brain directly.[9]

Caroline's case provided one of the most striking illustrations of this use. She was also a patient of Ost in our center for complementary medicine. At 28, she had just had surgery for an aggressive cancer of the stomach. The day after the operation, she was still in a great deal of pain. Only morphine, with which she dosed herself according to her need, gave her relief. However, her tolerance for the medication was low. Morphine made her confused and sometimes gave her violent nightmares. She needed an alternative, and quickly.

Ost had the opportunity to take care of her as part of a research program we were conducting at that time. At the beginning of her treatment, Caroline was so absorbed with her pain that she hardly noticed the three fine needles Thomas inserted in her hand, her leg, and her abdomen, adjusting them for 45 minutes. However, by the next day, she was scarcely using morphine anymore—only three small doses in 24 hours, according to the nurses' records. Two days later, she announced that the pain had almost entirely vanished. Also, she felt stronger and more determined than ever to get the better of her disease and not to let the doctors' pessimism get to her. Her anxiety seemed to have dissolved along with the

pain, without any of the typical side effects of morphinelike pain-
killers.*[10]

The Harvard study shows that acupuncture needles are, in fact,
able to block the regions of the emotional brain that are responsible
for the experience of pain and anxiety. This research helps us understand results as surprising as Caroline's. The research on rabbits that
no longer feel pain, in addition to studies of heroin addicts during
withdrawal, also suggest that acupuncture stimulates the secretion of
endorphins. These tiny molecules produced by the brain act like
morphine or heroin.

Researchers are beginning to discern a third mechanism: A session
of acupuncture seems to have a direct effect on the balance between
the two branches of the autonomic nervous system. It apparently increases activity of the parasympathetic system—the physiological
"brake"—at the expense of the sympathetic system—"the accelerator."
Thus, acupuncture promotes coherence in cardiac rhythm.[11]

Overall, acupuncture helps foster a return to equilibrium of the
autonomic nervous system. As we have seen in preceding chapters,
the roles of this equilibrium in emotional well-being, physical
health, slowing down of the aging process, and aversion of sudden
death have been reported in such prominent journals as the *Lancet*,
the *American Journal of Cardiology*, and *Circulation*. Does this physiological balance correspond to the equilibrium of "vital energy," the
"Qi," which the 2,500-year-old texts refer to? It probably is not pos-

---

*Several controlled studies record the benefits of acupuncture in reducing postoperative pain. On av-
erage, a daily session of acupuncture in the days following surgery can reduce doses of narcotics to
one-third of their usual amounts and thus limit side effects substantially. The best-known example
of that use was provided by the famous *New York Times* columnist James Reston. While he was in Beijing with President Nixon, Reston had to have an emergency appendectomy. After the "Western-
style" surgery, which saved his life, Reston suffered terribly from abdominal pain. He asked for
narcotics, but instead, they offered him two needles—one in his hand and the other in his tibia—
which he hardly felt. He was all the more surprised to discover, a few hours later, that his pain had
vanished. He was so struck by that experience that as soon as he got back to New York he published
a long article entitled, "Now, Let Me Tell You about My Appendectomy in Peking," in the *New York
Times* July 26, 1971. Overnight, Reston had opened the doors of America to acupuncture.

sible to reduce the Qi to a single function, but, to my thinking, the balance of the autonomic nervous system is certainly one of its facets. We know that meditation can influence this autonomic balance, as we saw in chapter 3. Nutrition can, too, as we shall see in the next chapter, and so can acupuncture. These three approaches are exactly what Chinese and Tibetan medical traditions have been recommending to influence the "Qi."

At the beginning of the 21st century, we are witnesses to unprecedented exchanges among medical and scientific cultures the world over. Like a new "Northwest Passage" across the Bering Strait, a bridge seems to have been laid between the great medical traditions of the West and the East. Functional imaging and the progress of molecular biology are beginning to help us understand the relations between the brain, the molecules of emotions (like endorphins), the balance of the autonomic nervous system, and the "flow of vital energy" the Ancients talked about. From these manifold connections a new physiology will probably emerge. Some, like Candice Pert, Ph.D., professor of physiology and biophysics at Georgetown University in Washington, D.C., call it the physiology of the "unified mind-body system."[12]

Acupuncture is only one of the three pillars of traditional Chinese and Tibetan medicine. The two others are physiological control through mental attitude—whether through meditation or the exercises in cardiac coherence discussed earlier—and nutrition. The wisdom of this medicine is becoming increasingly clear to our Western eyes. But, to traditional Asian practitioners, it would be senseless to use acupuncture or to cultivate our mental and physiological balance without paying special attention to the components that are constantly renewing our body—the food we take in. And yet nutrition is a field almost entirely abandoned by today's psychiatrists and psychotherapists. At the same time, very important discoveries have been made on the way nutrition contributes to the management of stress, anxiety, and depression—discoveries that can be put to use immediately.

9

The Revolution in Nutrition: Omega-3
Fatty Acids Feed the Emotional Brain

Patricia was 30 when her second son was born, just a year after her first one. Her partner, Jacques, was proud and happy. Over the previous year with their first child, their domestic life had been a succession of small blessings, and they had deeply desired this second infant. But now Jacques was surprised; Patricia didn't seem very happy. She was even moody and easily upset, taking little interest in the baby, seeking solitude, and sometimes breaking down in tears for no apparent reason. Even the breastfeeding that she had loved with her first baby now felt like a hardship.

Patricia had the "baby blues"—postpartum depression. About 1 young mother out of 10 experiences this condition, which is all the more alarming because it crowds out the happiness commonly anticipated with the birth of a child.[1] The baby was perfect, Jacques's restaurant was increasingly successful—so why was she so unhappy? Neither he nor Patricia could understand this sudden sadness. The doctors tried to reassure them with talk of "hormonal changes" that go along with pregnancy and especially childbirth itself, but that explanation did not really help.

In the last 10 years, an entirely new perspective on Patricia's problem has opened up. She lived in New York, where the daily consumption of one of the most important foods for the brain, the essential "omega-3" fatty acids, is particularly low, just as it is in the United Kingdom, in France, and in Germany.[2] These fatty acids, which the body itself cannot make (hence the term "essential"), play a major role in building the brain and maintaining its balance. That's why these fats are the principal nourishment the fetus takes in through the placenta. And that is also why the mother's reserves, which are already low in our Western-world diets, drop dramatically in the last weeks of pregnancy.

After birth, the omega-3 fatty acids continue to pass through to the baby via the mother's milk, of which they are one of the major components. Breastfeeding thus further depletes the mother's supply for her own body. If a second birth comes in the wake of a first one, as was Patricia's case, and if her diet in the meanwhile has remained poor in fish and shellfish, the principal source of these fatty acids, the mother is at substantial risk of depression.[3]

The "baby blues" occur between three and twenty times more frequently in the United States, France, and Germany than in Japan, Singapore, and Malaysia. According to the *Lancet*, these figures correspond to the differences between the Western and Asian countries with regard to the consumption of fish and shellfish; they can't be attributed simply to the tendency of Asians to hide their symptoms of depression.[4] If Jacques and Patricia had lived in Asia rather than the United States, her second experience of pregnancy and childbirth may have been very different. Understanding why is critical.

Brain Fuel

The brain is part of the body. Just like all the cells of all other organs, brain cells are continually being renewed. Tomorrow's cells are therefore made up of what we eat today.

One key neurological fact is that two-thirds of the brain is composed of fatty acids. These fats are the basic component of nerve cell membranes, the "envelope" through which all communications with other nerve cells take place, both within the brain and with the rest of the body. The food we eat is directly integrated into these membranes and makes up their substance. If we consume large quantities of saturated fats—such as butter or animal fat, which are solid at room temperature—their rigidity is reflected in the rigidity of the brain cells; if, on the other hand, we take in mostly polyunsaturated fats—those which are liquid at room temperature—the nerve cells' sheaths are more fluid and flexible and communication between them is more stable. Especially when those polyunsaturated fats are omega-3 fatty acids.[5]

The effects of these nutrients on behavior are striking. When omega-3 fatty acids are eliminated from the diet of laboratory rats, the animals' behavior radically changes in a few weeks. They become anxious, stop learning new tasks, and panic in stressful situations, such as seeking an escape route from a water pool.[6] Perhaps even more serious is the fact that a diet low in omega-3 reduces the capacity for pleasure. Much larger doses of morphine are required in these same rats to arouse them, despite the fact that morphine is the very model of easy gratification.[7]

On the other hand, a team of European researchers has shown that a diet rich in omega-3— such as the Eskimo's, consisting of up to 16 grams a day of fish oil[8]—leads, in the long run, to the increased production of neurotransmitters for energy and positive mood in the emotional brain.[9]

The fetus and the newborn child, with their rapidly developing brains, have the greatest need for omega-3 fatty acids. A recent Danish study published in the *British Medical Journal* shows that women who take in more omega-3 in their everyday diet during pregnancy have heavier and healthier infants, as well as fewer premature births.[10] Another Danish study, published this time in the

Journal of the American Medical Association, demonstrates that children who were breastfed for at least 9 months and who also received a great quantity of omega-3 in their diet have a higher IQ than others 20 or 30 years later.[11] And women in countries with the highest consumption of fish and the highest omega-3 levels in their breast milk are also considerably less likely to suffer from post-partum depression.[12] But the role of omega-3 is by no means limited to pregnancy.

Benjamin's Dangerous Energy

At first, Benjamin didn't know what was wrong with him. As the head of the biochemical laboratory of a large multinational pharmaceutical firm, he had always had exceptional reserves of energy. At 35, he had never experienced any problems with his health. Now he felt tired and listless. He first thought it might be a lingering cold—but this was no simple viral infection.

As soon as he arrived at his office, he would shut the door and avoid the company of his coworkers. He had even asked his assistant to cancel several important appointments on the pretext that he was too busy. As time went on, his behavior became increasingly strange. The meetings that he could not avoid made him extremely ill at ease. He felt incompetent and exposed. He found everybody else better informed, more creative, more dynamic than he was. He convinced himself that it was only a matter of time before his inadequacies would be revealed.

Once alone back in his office, he sometimes shut the door and cried, all the while telling himself that it was ridiculous to get so worked up. He expected to be dismissed from one day to the next and wondered what he would say to his wife and children.

Finally, because Benjamin was a doctor and the firm he worked for produced a commonly prescribed antidepressant, he decided to prescribe the medicine for himself. Barely 2 weeks later, he already felt much better. He went back to his usual routine, convinced that the worst was over. In fact, he was on the brink of disaster.

The medication seemed highly effective, but there were still some fluctuations in his condition from time to time, so Benjamin doubled the dose. And the drug seemed to work even better. Now, he was sleeping, at most, 4 hours a night and he was able to make up for the time that had been wasted over the previous months. He felt elated and he amused his colleagues with his slightly off-color jokes. One evening, when he stayed at work late with a young assistant, she leaned over his desk to pick up a file. He noticed that she wasn't wearing a bra, and he suddenly felt an overpowering attraction to her. He put his hand on hers. She yielded. That night, Benjamin didn't go home.

This dreary incident of sexual harassment would scarcely be original if it weren't for the fact that it was soon repeated with a laboratory employee and then, shortly afterwards, with a secretary. Benjamin had such a strong sexual drive that it was inconceivable for him to try to keep it under control. He didn't give a thought to its effect on the members of his staff. But soon, his advances started to become unwelcome to the women around him at work. And above all, as always happens in such circumstances, these women didn't really feel free to say "no."

Benjamin's misbehavior didn't stop there. He had become irritable, and his wife, who was beginning to feel frightened, no longer had the ability to influence him. He had forced her to sign a bank loan so that he could buy a sports car, then invested all their savings in disastrous operations on the stock market. But Benjamin's reputation and his productivity on the job were so respected that nobody dared speak out. At least, not yet.

His professional life started to fall apart the day one of his colleagues had had enough of his sexual advances and sexist comments. After a long battle with the firm—which wanted to keep Benjamin at all costs—his colleague's damaging testimony brought about the end of his brilliant career—and of his marriage. He was devastated, but Benjamin still had a long period of suffering ahead of him.

Once he had his back to the wall, Benjamin was willing to see a psychiatrist, whose diagnosis was beyond question. Benjamin was suffering from bipolar disorder, characterized by altering between periods of depression and "manic" phases, during which he lost his bearings to such an extent that his moral and financial judgments were dictated by a hedonistic need for instant gratification. These manic phases are often first set off by an antidepressant.

As soon as he stopped the medicine and took a tranquilizer, Benjamin's mood and his excess energy calmed down. Nevertheless, deprived of the artificial wind that had filled his sails, he awoke to the dramatic reality of his altered circumstances and became depressed again. This time, he certainly had good reason to feel sorry for himself.

For months, then years, he tried different medications that only succeeded in plunging him back into mania or depression. Besides, he was highly sensitive to the side effects of these drugs. He put on weight and felt "slowed down" almost to the point of exhaustion, even on standard doses of the mood stabilizers that were successively prescribed. The antidepressants that he took prevented him from sleeping and immediately affected his judgment again. Because of his history of illness, which was known in his profession, and his ongoing battle with depression, he couldn't find work, and he lived on his disability insurance. But everything changed the day when his psychiatrist, desperately seeking a breakthrough, suggested he try a treatment described in a study published by the principal periodical of experimental psychiatry: the *Archives of General Psychiatry*.

Benjamin, who was no longer taking any medication and who continued to suffer bouts of crying several times a week from no apparent cause, agreed unhesitatingly to take nine capsules a day of fish-oil extract—three before each of his three daily meals. This new tactic was a turning point. In a few weeks, his depression had vanished completely. Even more striking, in the course of the following year, was the fact that he had only one period of a few days during which he felt overenergetic.

Two years after the start of this treatment, Benjamin still takes no other medication than his fish-oil capsules. He has not yet reunited with his wife or daughters, but he has started working in a former colleague's laboratory. He is so talented that I have no doubt that he will make a comeback in his professional field in the coming years.

At Harvard, Andrew Stoll, M.D., was the first to prove the efficacy of using omega-3 fish oils in stabilizing mood swings and treating depression in manic-depressives. In the group he used for his study, only one patient had a relapse. The results were so convincing that researchers stopped conducting the study after only 4 months. The "control" group patients—those who got an olive oil placebo—relapsed at an astoundingly higher rate than those in the omega-3 group. Depriving the control group of omega-3 any longer could have been a breach of medical ethics.[13]

Having spent years studying the mechanisms of mood and depression, Dr. Stoll was so impressed by omega-3's effects that he wrote a book, *The Omega-3 Connection*, presenting his discoveries.[14] Since then, findings have shown that the benefits of omega-3 go beyond treating manic-depression.

Electroshocks vs. Fish Oil

Keith's parents seriously started to worry when his teachers suggested that he should abandon his studies because they felt that he could no longer concentrate enough to function in the class. Keith, with his soft features and his sharp intelligence, had not been completely well for more than 5 years. However, his parents had blamed this lack of focus on a difficult and perhaps unusually long adolescence.

In spite of his shyness and his periods of brooding, Keith had always been a good student. He was also very close to his mother and he enjoyed being with her. But, in the last few months, he had started refusing to eat in the school's cafeteria. He was uncomfortable in front of so many people he did not really know. Then he started to have anxiety attacks when he had to take the subway or get on a bus. His supposed "cowardice" made him very angry at himself, but he felt completely helpless when anxiety overwhelmed him. And he worried a bit more every week.

Soon, Keith started having trouble sleeping, which gave him less and less energy during the day, and his concentration became impaired. His grades started slipping and he was falling seriously behind.

As Keith had always counted on his schoolwork to shore up his fragile self-esteem, he now felt lost and started thinking about suicide. For 2 years, he was treated unsuccessfully with a whole range of antidepressants and anti-anxiety medications. When these did not work, his doctors had even tried an antipsychotic medication, normally used for schizophrenia. Adding lithium to his antidepressant for as long as 2 months did not help either. Finally, on the advice of Keith's psychiatrist, his mother took him to Basant Puri, M.D., Ph.D., a specialist of psychopharmacology at the Hammersmith Hospital in London.

Dr. Puri was very worried about the severity of Keith's symptoms. Keith's score on a standard measure of depression was the highest he had ever seen. Moreover, Keith now openly talked about committing suicide. He did so with uncanny detachment—as if it were the only and most obvious solution to his suffering—that made Dr. Puri shiver when listening to him. "Since I have to die someday anyhow," he said, "why wait any longer? Why should I suffer like this much more?"

And as Dr. Puri tried to argue his point, Keith interrupted him: "Let me die. Please. Out of charity."

After all the failed treatments, his new psychiatrist knew that only one intervention had a chance of overcoming such a deep and prolonged bout of depression: electroshock treatments. But Keith and his mother adamantly refused.

Dr. Puri took stock of the situation. Given the severity of Keith's condition, it was perfectly justified to hospitalize him against his will and that of his mother. It was also justified to submit him to electroshock treatments, in his own best interest, since practically every other treatment had already been tried. Time was running out to protect Keith from his self-destructive urges. Dr. Puri was getting ready to pursue this course of action when another, distant possibility came to his mind.

As Keith had not responded to any treatment, Dr. Puri thought, perhaps there was something defective in the very constituents of his nervous system. Dr. Puri remembered the intriguing results of a study, to which he had contributed, of omega-3 fatty acids in schizophrenia. In that study, the patient's depressive symptoms had improved significantly. He also remembered reading Dr. Stoll's book and learning about his results with bipolar patients.

With these thoughts in mind, Dr. Puri offered a deal to his young patient. He explained to him that he had reasons to believe that a new treatment, based on purified fish oils, might help him. Benefits remained very uncertain since, to his knowledge, Keith might be the first patient with a severe and chronic depression to be treated with fish oils. However, if Keith could promise that he would not try to harm himself, under any circumstances, for the next 2 months, and if he could promise to remain under the constant supervision of his mother, he, Dr. Puri, would be willing to take the risk of putting the electroshocks on hold for the time being, and trying the new treatment instead. Keith agreed.

The psychiatrist eliminated all of Keith's medications except for the last antidepressant Keith had been taking for 10 months. He then added a few grams per day of a purified fish oil, with the aim of regenerating Keith's neural membranes.

The results were spectacular. In a few weeks, the suicidal thoughts that had haunted Keith continuously for months disappeared completely. His discomfort in public places also vanished, and he started to sleep soundly again. Nine months later, all the symptoms of his 7-year depression had disappeared. His score on the severity of depression scale was now *zero*.

In addition to being a psychiatrist, Dr. Puri is a mathematician and a researcher in functional brain imaging. The Hammersmith Hospital in London is also one of the leading research centers in this field. Before treating Keith, he had obtained several MRI scans of his brain. When the same tests were repeated 9 months later, they revealed a completely different picture. The membranes of Keith's neurons appeared strengthened, and they no longer showed any evidence of leaking valuable constituents. The very structure of Keith's brain had been modified.

Keith's mother was delighted. Her son, the one she knew and whose loss she'd mourned, was back, transformed. Dr. Puri was so impressed by this transformation that he published a detailed description of the case in the *Archives of General Psychiatry*. He also initiated a multicenter study—as yet unfinished as I write these lines—on the effect of the fish oil extract on one of the most severe and deadly of all brain illnesses: Huntington's disease.[15]

In medicine, it is important to remain wary of what scientists call an "anecdote," a story of a singular, specific patient's treatment. We must refrain from building a theory or from widely recommending a treatment on the basis of a single case, or even a few, as extraordinary as they may seem. In order to truly prove its effectiveness, every promising treatment needs to submit to what is called a "randomized placebo-controlled study"—it must be compared to a placebo in a study in which neither patients nor physicians know who is receiving the active treatment and who is receiving a placebo.

Luckily, a few months after the publication of Keith's case by Dr. Puri, just such a study was published in the *American Journal of Psychiatry*. In Israel, Boris Nemets, M.D., and his colleagues at the Ben Gurion University of the Negev, studied a group of patients who, just like Keith, had been resistant to a range of antidepressant treatments. Dr. Nemets compared the efficacy of the same extract of purified fish oil—ethyl-eicosapentaenoic acid, or EPA—to an equivalent dose of olive oil (which, in spite of its antioxidant properties, does not contain any omega-3 fatty acids). More than half of the patients, who had not responded to their medications until then, saw their depression lessen dramatically in less than 3 weeks. Thus, Dr. Puri's anecdotal observation was confirmed. Since then, another study, from the United Kingdom, has been published, again in the *Archives of General Psychiatry*, which reaches the same conclusions. The study shows, in addition, that the entire range of depressive symptoms improves with omega-3 fatty acids: sadness as well as fatigue, anxiety as well as insomnia, decreased libido as well as any persistent thoughts that life is not worth living. Still another study, again from Harvard, and again in the *American Journal of Psychiatry*, also found that in young women who are "extremely moody," "often feel out of control," and find relationships "painful and difficult," an omega-3 supplement helped reduce depressive symptoms, as well as aggressive attitudes.[16]

We will probably need to wait for several years before enough studies of this type have been done to convince conventional psychiatrists of the potential benefits of omega-3 fatty acids. One confounding factor: Fish oils or flax seeds are natural products, and as such, they cannot be patented. Because of this simple economic fact, they are not of much interest to the large pharmaceutical companies that pay for the majority of the scientific studies of depression.

In the meantime, a number of other studies have suggested an important link between omega-3 fatty acids and depression. For example, depressed patients have lower stores of omega-3 fatty acids in their body than normal subjects.[17] And, the smaller their reserves are, the more severe their symptoms tend to be.[18] Even more striking, when patients who suffer from depression have more omega-3 fatty acids in their diet, their symptoms tend to be less impairing than those of depressed patients whose diet is deficient.[19] This goes along with a large study in Finland published in the *Archives of General Psychiatry* showing that frequent fish consumption (more than twice per week) is associated with lower risk for depression and decreased thoughts of life not being worth living in the general population.[20] And a 2003 population study in the Netherlands also confirmed that people over 60 years of age whose blood tests reveal higher levels of omega-3 fatty acids in their body are less likely to be depressed.[21]

The First Diet of <u>Homo Sapiens</u>

To understand this mysterious effect of omega-3 fatty acids on the brain and emotional balance, it may be necessary to go back to the origins of humanity. There are two types of "essential fatty acids": omega-3s and omega-6s. Omega-3s come from algae, plankton, and some leaves, including grass. Omega-6s come primarily from grains and abound in most vegetable oils and in animal fat, especially in the meat of animals fed with grains. Though omega-6s are also important constituents of cells, when present in excess they provoke inflammation responses throughout the body that can lead to a multitude of problems (we will return to this below).

At the time when the modern human brain developed, the early humanoids lived around the lakes of the Great Rift in East Africa. Scientists now believe that their food supply was perfectly balanced, with a ratio of 1-to-1 of omega-3s and omega-6s. This ideal ratio would have provided their bodies with the perfect building blocks for new kinds of neurons that developed new abilities such as self-consciousness, language, and the usage of tools.[22]

Today, the widespread development of certain livestock industry practices, including feeding livestock with grain rather than grass, in addition to the presence of omega-6-rich vegetable oil in all types of processed foods, has created a marked imbalance between omega-6s and omega-3s. The typical ratio of 3s to 6s in the Western diet is 1-to-10 to 1-to-20.[23] Some nutritionists have described our brains today as sophisticated race car engines meant to run on highly refined fuel that are instead asked to putter along on diesel.[24]

That mismatch between what the brain needs and what we feed it in America and in Europe would explain, in part, the large differences in the rates of depression between Western and Asian countries. In places such as Taïwan, Hong Kong, or Japan—where fish and seafood consumption is the highest—the rates of depression are considerably lower than in the United States. This remains true even after taking into account cultural differences that may effect self-disclosure of depressive symptoms.[25] The mismatch may have also contributed to the rapid growth of depression in the West over the last 50 years. Today, the consumption of omega-3 fatty acids in the Western diet may be less than half of what it was before World War II.[26] And it is precisely since that period that rates of depression have risen considerably.[27]

An excess of omega-6s in the body leads to inflammation reactions.[28] One of the more striking developments in recent medical research is the revelation that all of the leading illnesses in the Western world are caused or worsened by inflammatory reactions: cardiovascular diseases—such as coronary artery disease, myocardial infarctions, or strokes—but also cancer, arthritis, and even Alzheimer's disease.[29] And there is a striking overlap between countries with the highest rates of cardiovascular diseases[30] and those

with the highest rates of depression.[31] This does, indeed, suggest
the possibility of common causes for both. And, in fact, omega-3s
have well-established benefits for cardiac diseases, known for a
much longer time than those that have just been studied with respect to depression.

One of the first large studies on omega-3s and cardiovascular diseases was done in Lyon, the capital of French gastronomy, by researchers Serge Renaud, Ph.D., of the University of Bordeaux and
Michel de Lorgeril, M.D., of the University of Grenoble. In an article published in the *Lancet*, they showed that cardiac patients who followed a "Mediterranean diet" rich in omega-3 fatty acids had a 76
percent lower chance of dying in the 2 years following their myocardial infarction than those who followed the diet recommended by
the American Heart Association.[32] Several other studies also document how omega-3 fatty acids strengthen heart rate variability and
protect the heart against arrhythmias.[33] As we saw in chapter 3, more
heart rate variability is also associated with less anxiety and depression. It is therefore conceivable that depression and cardiovascular
illnesses both increase together in societies with a strong imbalance
in the omega-3-to-omega-6 ratio in the diet.

Is Depression Inflammation?

The discovery of the important role of omega-3 fatty acids in the prevention and treatment of depression raises entirely new questions
about the nature of this disorder. What if depression were an inflammatory disease, as we now know is the case for coronary artery disease, the leading cause of death in Western societies? An inflammation
theory of depression may begin to explain a number of puzzling
observations about this disease that most contemporary theories—entirely focused on neurotransmitters such as serotonin—have been
dutifully ignoring.

Take the situation of Nancy, for example. She was 65 when she experienced her first episode of depression. Nothing had changed in her life, and she just could not understand why she would suddenly become depressed. Yet, her family doctor pointed out that she had symptoms of sadness and hopelessness, lack of energy, fatigue, impaired concentration, no appetite, and even weight loss. All of these were, he insisted, typical symptoms of depression and met the diagnostic criteria for major depressive disorder of the American Psychiatric Association.

Six months later, before she had even agreed to start treatment for her depression, Nancy noticed a persistent pain in her stomach. The ultrasound that her doctor ordered revealed a large tumor on the edge of her liver. Nancy had pancreatic cancer. As is often the case in this illness, her cancer had manifested first with a depression rather than with physical symptoms. Several types of cancer induce widespread inflammatory reactions well before the tumor becomes large enough for detection. That inflammatory state, which is sometimes subtle, may well be responsible for the symptoms of depression that precede the diagnosis of cancer. In fact, depression is common in all physical illnesses that have a diffuse inflammatory component, such as infections (pneumonia, the flu, typhoid fever), cerebrovascular accidents ("strokes"), myocardial infarctions, and autoimmune disorders. I wonder, therefore, to what extent "classic" depressions may also be caused by inflammatory processes. That would not be much of a surprise, since we know that stress in and of itself causes inflammatory reactions— which is the reason why it also worsens acne, arthritis, and most autoimmune diseases.[34] Since a long period of stress often precedes depression, it may well be that depressive symptoms are caused directly by stress-related inflammation. In the end, Tibetan medicine may be right: Depression is perhaps as much a physical illness as it is a disorder of the mind.

Where Can You Find Omega-3 Essential Fatty Acids?

The primary sources of omega-3 fatty acids are algae and plankton. These find their way to our kitchens and plates through fish and seafood that accumulate the fatty acids in their fat tissue. Cold water fish—richer in fat—are therefore the best sources of omega-3s. Farm-raised fish may be less rich in omega-3s than fish from the wild. Ocean-fished salmon, for example, is an excellent source of omega-3s, but farm-raised salmon is not as reliable.*

The most reliable sources of omega-3s, and the least contaminated by mercury, dioxin, and organic carcinogens, are the smaller fish, because they're found at the bottom of the food chain. These are mackerel (one of the richest sources of omega-3s), anchovies (whole, not the small salted fillets found on pizza), sardines, and herring. Other good fish sources of omega-3s are tuna, haddock, and trout.[†] (See the table, "Good Sources of Omega-3s," on page 139.)

Good vegetarian sources of omega-3s also exist, though they require one more step in metabolism to become actual constituents of neural membranes. These are flax seeds (which can be eaten as such, ground, or slightly roasted), flaxseed oil,[‡] canola (rapeseed) oil, hemp oil, and English walnuts. All green leafy vegetables contain precursors of omega-3 fatty acids, though in lesser amounts. One of the best vegetable sources is purslane (a basic staple of Roman cooking 2,000 years ago, and still commonly used in modern Greece). Omega-3s

---

*It is difficult to precisely rate the omega-3 content of farm-raised fish, as each farm uses its own blend for the fish's diet, which is where the essential fatty acids come from. In his very thorough book on omega-3 fatty acids, Dr. Stoll suggests that European farms have stricter standards for fish food than American farms. According to him, the omega-3 content of European farm-raised fish is comparable to that of fish from the wild. (A. Stoll, *The Omega-3 Connection*, 2001)

[†]Shark and swordfish are also rich in omega-3, but they are often contaminated with mercury to such an extent that the FDA advises pregnant women and young children to avoid them altogether. (FDA Consumer Advisory, www.cfsan.fda.gov/~dms/admehg.html)

[‡]Flaxseed oil can become toxic if it is not refrigerated and protected from light. It is therefore essential to purchase freshly pressed oil that has been continuously refrigerated and stored in an opaque container. The oil should never taste excessively bitter (even if by nature it is mildly bitter).

GOOD SOURCES OF OMEGA-3s

FOOD ITEM	AMOUNT OF OMEGA-3
100 g (3.5 ounces) of mackerel	2.5 g
100 g (3.5 ounces) of herring	1.7 g
100 g (3.5 ounces) of tuna (even canned)	1.5 g (except if low-fat tuna, of course, from which the omega-3s have been eliminated)
100 g (3.5 ounces) of whole anchovies	1.5 g
100 g (3.5 ounces) of salmon	1.4 g
100 g (3.5 ounces) of sardines	1 g
Flax seeds (which can be eaten as such, ground, or slightly roasted), 1 tablespoon	2.8 g
Flaxseed oil, 1 tablespoon	7.5 g
Canola (rapeseed) oil, 1 tablespoon	1.3 g
English walnuts, 1 cup	2.3 g
Purslane, 1 cup	457 mg
Spinach, 1 cup	384 mg
Seaweeds (dried), 1 tablespoon	268 mg
Spirulina, 1 tablespoon	260 mg
Watercress, 1 cup	528 mg

can also be derived from spinach, seaweeds, and spirulina (a traditional part of the Aztec diet).

The meat of wild or farm animals that feed on grass and natural
leaves also contains omega-3s. For this reason, wild game is generally much richer in omega-3s than livestock (at least nonorganic
livestock).[35] The more grain livestock is fed, the lower the omega-3
content of its flesh. A report published in the *New England Journal of
Medicine* shows, for example, that the eggs of free-range chickens
contain 20 times more omega-3s than those of grain-fed hens.[36] The
meat of grain-fed livestock also becomes richer in omega-6s, with
their *pro*-inflammatory properties. Therefore, in order to maintain a
balance between omega-3s and omega-6s, it is important to limit
meat consumption to a maximum of three servings per week, and to
avoid fatty meats, even those richer in omega-6s, and saturated fats
that compete with omega-3s.

All vegetable oils are rich in omega-6s and none contain omega-
3s, except flaxseed oil, canola (rapeseed) oil, and hemp oil, each of
which is at least one-third omega-3. (Flaxseed oil is more than 50 percent omega-3s, making it the best vegetable source of these essential
fatty acids.) Olive oil can be used freely; it does not contain many
omega-3s or omega-6s, so it does not affect the ratio. To approach an
omega-3-to-omega-6 ratio as close as possible to 1-to-1, you should
aim to eliminate almost all the usual cooking oils, except for olive oil
and canola (rapeseed) oil. Avoiding frying oil is particularly important; in addition to its omega-6 content, frying oil has many free rad-
icals that produce oxidative reactions inside the body.

Butter, cream, and full-fat dairy products should be eaten with mod-
eration because they compete with omega-3s for integration within
cells. Yet, Serge Renaud, who conducted research on cheese and yo-
gurt in France, has demonstrated that these products—even made from
whole milk—are much less toxic than other milk products because
their high calcium and magnesium content reduces the absorption of
saturated fats.[37] This is the reason why Artemis Simopoulos, M.D.,

former chair of the Nutrition Coordinating Committee at the National Institutes of Health, considers that up to 30 grams of cheese per day are acceptable in her "Omega Diet Plan."[38] In addition, some new and intriguing studies suggest that dairy products, eggs, and even meat derived from animals fed in part with flax seeds—about 5 percent of the animals' diet—may help reduce cholesterol as well as insulin resistance in type 2 diabetes.[39] These products may become a very important source of omega-3s in the future.

The findings from existing studies suggest that in order to obtain an antidepressant effect, one must consume between 1 and 10 grams per day of the combination of DHA (docosahexaenoic acid) and EPA (eicosapentaenoic acid)—the two forms of omega-3s commonly found in fish oil. In practice, many people opt for an omega-3 supplement in order to be sure they're receiving a sufficiently pure, reliable, and quality "dosage" of the nutrient. Several products are available from supplement manufacturers, in the form of either capsules or oil. The best products are probably those that have the highest concentration of EPA with respect to DHA. Some authors, such as Dr. Stoll and David Horrobin, M.D., Ph.D., former chair of medicine at the University of Montreal, suggest that it is mostly EPA that has an antidepressant effect and that too much DHA may actually block the effect, requiring higher doses of the combined oil than if the product is more concentrated in EPA. Indeed, a study from the Baylor College of Medicine found that a pure DHA supplement had no effect against depression, which contrasts sharply with the results of studies using EPA.[40] Products with a very high EPA concentration (at least seven times more EPA than DHA) may require only 1 gram per day of EPA. This is the dose that was used in three studies that looked specifically at patients with depressive symptoms.

Products that contain a bit of vitamin E are better protected against oxidation, which may render the oil ineffective or even, in rare cases, toxic. Some doctors recommend combining an omega-3 supplement with a daily vitamin supplement that contains vitamin E (no more than

800 International Units per day), vitamin C (no more than 1,000 milligrams per day), and selenium (no more than 200 micrograms per day) to prevent oxidation of the omega-3 fatty acids inside the body. However, I did not find any evidence that this extensive supplementary regimen was truly necessary.[41]

Cod liver oil, a favorite of our grandparents as a source of vitamin A and D, is not a reliable long-term source of omega-3 fatty acids. Taking an adequate dose of cod liver oil for depression would require such large amounts that it might result in a dangerous overload of vitamin A.

Curiously, despite the fact that some patients balk at the idea of taking "fat" supplements, omega-3-based oils do not seem to make people gain weight. In his study of patients with bipolar illness, Dr. Stoll noted that patients did not gain weight in spite of their daily intake of 9 grams of fish oil. In fact, some even lost weight.[42] In a study performed with mice, those who were fed a diet particularly rich in omega-3s were 25 percent leaner than those who ate exactly the same amount of calories, but without omega-3s. Some authors have suggested that the way the body metabolizes omega-3s reduces the buildup of fat tissue.[43]

The only side effects from omega-3 supplements are fishy aftertaste (usually eliminated by taking the supplements in divided doses at the beginning of meals); occasional loose stools or mild diarrhea (which may require reducing the dose for a few days); and, in rare cases, bruising or increased bleeding time. People who are taking anticoagulant medicines such as Coumadin, or even a daily aspirin (which also increases bleeding time), should be careful not to take more than 1,000 milligrams per day of fish oil, and to consult their physician.

The Judgment of History

On the day historians begin to analyze the history of medicine in the 20th century, I believe they will point out two major events. The first one, without any doubt, was the discovery of antibiotics, which practically eradicated bacterial pneumonia—the leading cause of death in the West until World War II. The second is a revolution that is still in the making: the scientific demonstration that nutrition has a profound impact on practically all the leading causes of disease in Western societies.

Cardiologists and internists have been the first to integrate this fundamental idea into their practices (even if, to this day, they rarely recommend omega-3 diets or supplements, despite the large number of studies published in respected journals that have documented their effects, as well as the explicit recommendations of the American Heart Association[44]). Most psychiatrists lag far behind. Yet the brain is almost certainly as sensitive to the contents of our daily diets as the heart may be. When we regularly intoxicate our brain with alcohol or street drugs, it suffers. When we fail to nourish it with the nutrients it needs, it suffers, too. What's truly astonishing is that it's taken so long for modern Western science to come back to this very basic realization. All traditional medicines, whether Tibetan, Chinese, Ayurvedic, or Greco-Roman, have emphasized the importance of nutrition since their earliest texts. Hippocrates wrote: "Let your food be your treatment, and your treatment your food." That was 2,400 years ago.

But there is still another door to the emotional brain that relies entirely on the body. Hippocrates knew about it as well, and it has been ignored in the West, just as nutrition has. Curiously, this method is disparaged even more by people who suffer from stress or depression, with the pretext that they do not have enough time or enough energy. Yet, it is one of the most abundant sources of energy, and it has been well-substantiated by controlled studies. That door is physical exercise—even, as we will see, at low doses.

10

Prozac or Puma?

Bernard was a highly successful movie producer in his forties. He was tall and elegant, and his irresistible smile must have helped him gain the trust of others in his profession. Who wouldn't be won over by his charm? Yet, Bernard was at the end of his rope. Anxiety attacks had been poisoning his life for the past 2 years.

The first time he had an attack was at a power lunch in a packed restaurant. Everything was going along fine when Bernard suddenly felt sick. He became nauseated, his heart was beating wildly, and he could hardly breathe. The image of his childhood friend, who had been struck down by an infarction the year before, suddenly crossed his mind. With that thought, his heart started beating even faster, and he could not focus his thinking at all. His vision became clouded, and he could feel the people and the surroundings becoming strangely remote and unreal. In a flash, Bernard understood that this was it—he was dying.

He murmured a vague excuse to his associates and quickly headed toward the exit. Hailing a taxi, Bernard asked to be taken directly to the emergency room at the nearest hospital. Once he was checked in and had been examined, the doctors there assured him that he was not actually about to die. To the contrary, they explained, he had simply had an anxiety—or rather, a "panic"—attack.

One person out of every five who have this type of attack first goes to an emergency room, not to a psychiatrist (and almost half of them arrive by ambulance). In fact, over the next 2 years, Bernard spent a lot of time in the emergency ward, as well as at several cardiologists' offices. He was repeatedly assured that his symptoms had nothing to do with his heart. A tranquilizer, Xanax, was even prescribed, "to help you relax," they said.

The medication helped him at first. The attacks stopped and he started to increasingly rely on his little pill. He had even begun to take four a day, just to make sure the anxiety did not bother him in his work. Little by little, he noticed that if he was a bit behind in his dose, the anxiety was greater. One day when he was traveling, his luggage was stolen and, with it, his Xanax. After a few hours, his anxiety was so great and his heart started beating so strongly that he still describes that day as the worst one of his life. When he got home, he vowed to overcome his dependence on Xanax and never take it again.

A few years earlier, Bernard had noticed that if he swam for 30 minutes he would feel better for an hour or two. So, he took up swimming again, but the feeling of well-being did not last long enough. The "spinning" fad—indoor group bicycling—was all the rage, and one of Bernard's friends convinced him to try. Three times a week, he joined a dozen other people in a health club and swayed on a stationary bicycle to the frenetic pace their instructor imposed. Nobody was allowed to fall behind. The pulse of the techno music and emulation of the other cyclers encouraged him to keep up. At the end of the hour, he was both exhausted and in high spirits. That intense sensation of well-being lasted for hours.

In fact, Bernard soon discovered that it was best if he didn't cycle after seven or eight in the evening if he wanted to sleep that night. But the most astonishing result was that he gained a lot more confidence in his ability to deal with panic attacks. After a few weeks, the attacks ceased completely. Today, 2 years later, Bernard still talks about the amazing benefits of spinning to anybody who will listen. He still goes to classes at least three times a week, especially when he is under stress. He has not had an attack since.

Bernard freely admits that he is "hooked on spinning." If he stops exercising, he starts feeling out of sorts within a few days. When he travels, he never forgets his running shoes, so as to "let off steam," as he says. In any case, exercise is an addiction that does not just make him feel good—it also helps him keep his weight down, build up his libido, improve his sleep, reduce his blood pressure, and strengthen his immune system. It protects him against heart diseases and even against certain cancers. If he is truly "addicted," his addiction to exercise makes him feel that he has *more* control over his life—exactly the opposite of what had happened with Xanax.

A Treatment for Anxiety . . . and Immune Cells

Bernard is not alone. What he discovered on his own, Plato had described thousands of years ago. And in the course of the last 20 years, Western science has demonstrated it: Exercise is a remarkably effective treatment for anxiety.

Studies on this subject are now so numerous that there are even several "meta-analyses," or studies of studies.[1] One such study even specifically deals with the benefits of using a regular stationary bicycle, which is much less intense than the "spinning" Bernard is so fond of. This study shows that the majority of participants felt more energetic, as well as more relaxed, after using a stationary bike.[2] The benefits were still evident a year later, the research records show, as the vast majority of the participants had decided, on their own, to continue exercising regularly.

The curious thing is that the less fit we are—the richer our meals, the more time we spend in front of TV or behind the wheel of a car—the faster physical exercise, even in small doses, will make us feel better.[3] Turns out, Bernard was also right to increase his dose of exercise in periods of greater stress.

At the University of Miami, Arthur LaPerrière, Ph.D., examined the protective effect of exercise in difficult situations. For his test, he chose one of the most terrible moments a human being can experience—the one in which a person is told that he or she is HIV-positive. At the time of that research, long before the discovery of tritherapy, the diagnosis amounted to a death sentence. And people were left to deal psychologically with this devastating fact all alone.

Patients who had been exercising regularly for at least 5 weeks, Dr. LaPerrière observed, seemed to be "protected" against fear and despair. Moreover, their immune systems, which often collapse in stressful situations, also resisted better when they got the terrible news. "Natural killer" (NK) cells are the body's first line of defense against both outside invasion—like the AIDS virus—and the spread of cancer cells. They are highly sensitive to our emotions. The better we feel, the more energetically they do their job. On the other hand, in periods of stress and depression, these natural killer cells tend to abate or to stop multiplying. This outcome is exactly what Dr. LaPerrière observed in cases of patients who did not exercise. Their NK cells decreased abruptly after the diagnosis—just the opposite of patients who exercised regularly.[4]

The Initiation of Xaviera

A little jogging is also good for people with depression. In one of the first modern articles on the subject, John Greist, M.D., of the University of Wisconsin—Madison, tells Xaviera's story.

Xaviera was a 28-year-old student who was pursuing a second

master's at the University of Wisconsin. She lived alone, rarely went out except to her classes, and constantly complained that she would never meet the man of her life. Her existence seemed empty and she had lost hope that it would change.

Her only consolation was her beloved three packs of cigarettes a day. She spent her time watching them waft upwards in smoke wreaths, instead of concentrating on her course notes. She was not really surprised when the doctor at the school clinic told her that her score on a scale for depression placed her in a group with the most affected 10 percent of the patients there. By then, her depression had been going on for 2 years and none of the suggested treatments was acceptable to her.

Xaviera did not want to talk to a psychologist about her mother and her father or the problems of her childhood. She refused medication because, as she said, "I may be depressed, but I'm not sick." She nevertheless agreed to take part in a research project the doctor was conducting, perhaps because it was a challenge.

Xaviera was supposed to run three times a week for 20 to 30 minutes, alone or in a group, as she wished. At her first meeting with her jogging instructor, she wondered if it was a joke. How could he possibly expect a person 20 pounds overweight who had not exercised since the age of 14 and who smoked three packs of cigarettes a day to be a proper candidate for a study on jogging? The last time she had gone cycling she had lasted 10 minutes and thought she was going to die. She had sworn to herself, "Never again." And then the idea that she needed an *instructor* to learn how to run seemed even more ridiculous. What was there to learn? To walk fast putting one foot in front of the other?

Still, Xaviera listened to the advice her instructor gave her, and this guidance turned out to be absolutely essential to her future success. First, she was told to take very small steps, trotting rather than running, leaning forward very slightly, without raising her knees too much. Above all, she was told to go slowly enough to hold a conversation ("You have to be able to talk, but not sing," her instructor insisted). If she got out of breath, she was ordered to slow down—if need be, to no more than a brisk walking pace. She must never experience pain or fatigue.

The goal at the outset was simply to cover a mile, taking as much time as she liked, trying to jog as much as possible. The fact that she managed to reach this objective on the very first day was a source of satisfaction for her. After 3 weeks, at a rate of three weekly sessions, she was able to keep up her jogging pace for a mile and a half, then 2 miles without too much hardship. She had to admit that she was feeling a little better—overall, she was sleeping more soundly, feeling more energetic, and spending less time feeling sorry for herself.

Little by little, Xaviera made further progress, and every day over the 5-week period, she felt better. Then one day, she forced a bit too much at the end of her run and twisted her ankle—not enough to be completely immobilized, but enough to have to stop running for 3 weeks. A few days later, she was the first to be surprised at how disappointed she was not to be able to go jogging. Deprived of 1 week's jogging, she noticed that her symptoms of depression were starting to come back. Dark thoughts came crowding in, and she started feeling pessimistic about everything again.

However, when Xaviera finally went back to what had become "her" exercise, her symptoms waned once again within a few weeks. She had never felt so well. Even her period—which was usually so painful—seemed less uncomfortable. When she spoke to her coach after her first run in 3 weeks, she told him, "I'm out of shape, but I know that it will come back, and I definitely feel better than the first time I ran."

While we'll never know if she stopped smoking or met the man of her dreams, long after the research project ended, according to Dr.

Greist, Xaviera was still regularly spotted running around the lake with a smile on her face.[5]

The Runner's High

Depression is always associated with dark, pessimistic thoughts, thoughts that undercut the self and others and that turn relentlessly over in our heads: "I'll never succeed. Anyhow, it's not worth trying. It won't work. I'm ugly. I'm not intelligent enough. I have bad luck. This always happens to me. I don't have enough energy, strength, courage, willpower, ambition. I've really hit bottom. People don't like me. I don't have any talent. I don't deserve attention. I don't deserve to be loved. I'm sick. . . ."

These ideas may be as excessive as they are hurtful (such as, "I always disappoint everybody," which simply cannot be true). But by the time they are manifest in depression, these thoughts have usually become so automatic that it is no longer obvious how abnormal they are, just the outward sign of a sickness in the soul rather than an objective reality. Through his work, which began in the sixties and seventies, Aaron Beck, M.D., the inventor of cognitive therapy, has shown that simply repeating these thoughts in one's mind maintains depression. He also showed that deliberately stopping them often helps patients find their way back to well-being.[6]

One of the characteristics of sustained physical effort is precisely that it puts a halt, at least temporarily, to this torrent of depressive thoughts. Such thoughts rarely come up spontaneously during exercise. If they do, diverting your attention by fixing your thoughts on your breathing, or on the sensation of your feet pressing down on the ground, or on your awareness of your spinal column, is usually enough to see them off. Most people who jog or run say that after 15 or 20 minutes of sustained effort, they reach a state in which their thoughts are spontaneously positive and even creative. They are less conscious of themselves and let the rhythm of their effort guide and lead them on. This experience is what some refer to as the "runner's high." Only joggers who persevere for several weeks experience it. This state, subtle as it is (and it is a far cry from heroin), often becomes addictive. After a certain amount of consistent exercise, many joggers can no longer go without their 20 minutes of running, even for a single day.

The big mistake that beginners make when they come back from a store proudly sporting their new running shoes is to want to run too fast for too long. Truthfully, there is no magic speed or distance. What leads to a state of "flow" is perseverance in an effort that you sustain at the limit of your capacities. *At the limit*, but no further. Mikhail Csikszentmihalyi, Ph.D., the researcher on "states of flow," has demonstrated this brilliantly. For a beginner, the distance will inevitably be short and the steps small. Later, the runner may have to run faster and longer in order to maintain "flow," but only after he or she has probably already become addicted!

Zooming Past Zoloft

Researchers at Duke University have recently carried out a study comparing the antidepressant effects of jogging with those of Zoloft, a well-known and effective antidepressant. After 4 months, patients treated with either approach were doing equally well. The medication offered no particular advantage over the regular practice of jogging. Even combining the medicine and jogging at the same time did not enhance the effects. On the other hand, a year later, there was a major difference between the two types of treatment. More than a third of the patients who had been treated with Zoloft had relapsed, whereas 92 percent of those who had followed the jogging program were still doing well.[7] They had decided on their own initiative to keep on exercising even after the study had ended.

Another research project at Duke has shown that youth and good health are not necessary to get benefits from physical exercise. Depressed patients aged 50 to 77 benefited just as much from 30 minutes of brisk walking (without running) three times a week as they did from an antidepressant. The antidepressant relieved the symptoms a little faster, but not more effectively. That was the only difference.[8]

Regular physical exercise may not only heal an episode of depression, but can also probably help prevent one as well. In a population of normal subjects, people who were exercising at the beginning of the study were much less likely to experience depression during the next 25 years.[9]

I have experienced both the treatment and prevention effects of exercise in my own life. When, at 22, I first arrived in America, I hardly knew anybody. My first months were filled with all the usual orienting activities of immigrants. Besides my courses in medical school, which were very time consuming, I was looking for an apartment and moving in. Starting all over again without parents around to tell me what to do and how to do it was fun at the beginning. I remember the pleasure I took in the simple joy of buying curtains, or even a frying pan, for the first time. But after a few months, once I had settled in and was caught up in my study routine, my life seemed particularly empty, devoid of pleasures.

Without my family, my friends, my culture, my favorite "hangouts," I suddenly realized that I felt as if I were slowly withering away. I remember one evening in particular, nothing seemed to matter or make sense except classical music. I listened to it endlessly instead of delving into my studies. I even said to myself that conducting an orchestra was the only profession that might be worth practicing in such a cold and indifferent world.

As I did not have the slightest chance of succeeding in that profession, my pessimism as an isolated immigrant only got worse. After several weeks in this stark mood, I realized that if I did not react, I was going to fail my exams. Leaving France to come all the way to America just to fail would've been absurd—then I really would have a reason to be depressed!

I didn't know where to begin, but I knew I had to shake myself out of the stupor that left me sitting around for hours not doing anything except listening to the same tapes over and over. I thought about squash, which I had taken up in Paris before leaving. Luckily, I had even brought my racket with me—and it saved me.

First, I joined a squash club. During the first 2 weeks of playing, nothing changed, except that I finally had something pleasurable to look forward to in my life. I knew that at least three times a week I would enjoy expending my physical energy and then taking a long, well-deserved shower.

Thanks to squash, I also met a few people who were nice enough to invite me over for dinner. Little by little, I made friends and found a rewarding social life. For a long time, I did not know whether it was the exercise or my new friends that helped me most, but whatever the explanation, it didn't matter much. I felt far better, and I was back in the saddle.

Later, I learned that even in the most trying times, if I ran for 20 minutes at least every other day, usually alone, I was then much better equipped to handle challenges, and that I was able, in any case, to avoid the throes of depression. And despite all of the research and investigations that I've done, nothing that I've learned since has led me to change what is still my "first line of defense" against life's uncertainties.

Stimulating Pleasure

By what mysterious processes does exercise have such an impact on the emotional brain? Naturally, there is, first of all, its effect on endorphins. These tiny molecules secreted by the brain resemble opium and its derivatives, such as morphine and heroin. The emotional brain contains many receptors for endorphins,[10] and that's why it is so sensitive to opium—it immediately radiates a sensation of well-being and satisfaction by hijacking one of the emotional brain's own intrinsic mechanisms. Opium has a powerful effect on emotions—in fact, it's the strongest known antidote to the pangs of separation and mourning.[11]

However, when derivatives of opium are used too often, they can become habit forming. Brain receptors become inured to them, so the dose must be systematically increased in order to produce the same effect. Moreover, because the receptors become less and less sensitive, regular pleasures lose all their power and potency—including sex, the pleasure of which is often reduced to nothing in drug addicts.

The secretion of endorphins brought on by physical exercise does exactly the opposite. The more the natural mechanism of pleasure is gently stimulated by exercise, the more sensitive the mechanism itself becomes. In addition to relishing sex and life's other big pleasures, people who exercise regularly actually get *more* pleasure out of the little things in life: their friendships, their cats, their meals, their hobbies, or even the smiles of passersby in the street. Essentially, it becomes easier for them to be satisfied. And in fact, the experience of pleasure is just the opposite of depression. Depression is defined, above all, by the *absence of pleasure*, more so than by sadness, which is probably the reason why the release of endorphins has such a potent antidepressant and anxiolytic effect.[12]

Stimulating the emotional brain by these natural processes also kindles the immune system. It promotes the proliferation of those so-called "natural killer" cells, making them more aggressive against infections and cancer cells.[13] (See "Emotions Profoundly Influence Body Functions," page 156.) The opposite effect occurs with heroin addicts, whose immune defenses collapse, often causing them to become gravely ill.

Exercise may also strengthen another physiological mechanism related to emotional health. This mechanism involves what we have already learned about heart rate variability. People who

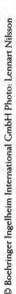

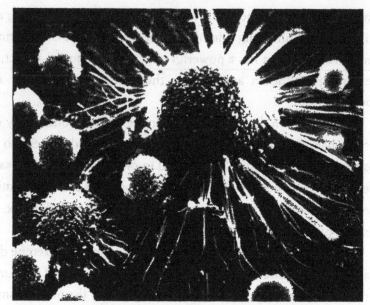

EMOTIONS PROFOUNDLY INFLUENCE BODY FUNCTIONS

"Natural killer" cells of the immune system are the first line of defense of the body. Like many other physiological functions, they are under the control of the emotional brain. Positive emotions such as peacefulness and well-being stimulate these cells. Stress, anxiety, and depression interfere with their function. Here, natural killer cells (smaller), are attacking a cancer cell (larger, in center).

exercise regularly show a greater variability in heart rate and more coherence than people who do not.[14] This means that their parasympathetic system, the physiological "brake" that brings on periods of calm, is healthier and stronger. A good balance between the two branches of the autonomic nervous system is one of the best potential antidotes to anxiety and panic attacks. All the symptoms of anxiety start with an overactive sympathetic system—a dry mouth, accelerated heartbeat, sweating, trembling, a rise in blood pressure. The sympathetic and parasympathetic systems are always in opposition. Thus, the more stimulation the parasympathetic branch receives, the stronger it becomes—like a developing muscle. When it is strong enough, it simply blocks the symptoms of anxiety.

A new treatment for depression is under experimentation in major centers for biological psychiatry around the world. A device implanted under the skin stimulates the parasympathetic system. Like bodybuilding machines that contract your abdominal muscles while you watch television, using a slight electric discharge, this treatment of the future requires no effort from the patient. It claims to be able to bring on the beneficial effects of the parasympathetic system. Several preliminary studies of patients whose previous treatments had failed make it seem very promising.[15] I personally think that physical exercise and the practice of cardiac coherence may produce exactly the same outcome, provided that patients are still motivated enough to undertake them.

The Keys to Success

Even when we're convinced that regular exercise matters, sometimes it seems like nothing can be harder to integrate into our daily lives— even more so when we're depressed or under stress. However, a few very simple secrets make it easier to undertake a more active physical life.

First of all, you do not have to get a lot of physical exercise; what's important is *regularity*. Various studies show that the minimum quantity needed to affect the emotional brain is 20 minutes of exercise three times a week. The duration seems to matter, but not the distance covered, nor the intensity of the effort. If you sustain the effort to the point where you can still talk but cannot sing, that's plenty.

As with certain medications, the benefits, on the other hand, may be in proportion to the "dose" of exercise. The more severe the symptoms of depression or anxiety, the more regular and intense the exercise required. Five sessions a week are better than three. An hour of spinning is more likely to be effective than 20 minutes of steady walking. Still, the worst scenario would be to try spinning, for example, get overly tired and out of breath, and then give up altogether. In this case, 20 minutes of regular walking would be vastly more effective.

Begin gently and let your body be your guide. The objective is to reach the state of flow Dr. Csikszentmihalyi describes. To do so, you must always be at the limit of your capacities and no further, as the limit of your capacities is the doorway to "flow." (Think of the talk-but-not-sing principle.) When your capacity expands, as a result of training, you will always have time to run farther and faster. And, curiously, the available research does not establish a distinction between "aerobic" exercise (such as running, swimming, bicycling, and tennis), which tends to produce shortness of breath and what is called "anaerobic" exercise (such as weight training). A thorough review in the *British Medical Journal* concludes that they are equally effective, at least with respect to depressive symptoms.[16]

To heighten the benefits, most studies suggest that group exercise is still more effective than individual practice. When a group is devoted to the same goal, the support and encouragement of others, or simply the example that these like-minded people set, can make a big difference. If nothing else, that group dynamic can motivate you on rainy days, when you are late, or when there is a good movie on TV. . . . Bottom line: People who exercise in groups abide more readily by the need for regularity that is so crucial to success.

Finally, you should choose a kind of exercise that is fun for you. The more it resembles a game, the easier it will be to stick to. Many companies have informal basketball teams or walking clubs that meet a few times a week for an hour at the end of the day. A volleyball team or tennis club can serve the same purpose, provided that the practice is regular. But if you love swimming and hate running, don't make yourself jog. You will probably not keep it up.

Here's a tip that several of my patients have found useful: You can get more fun out of your stationary bike, stair stepper, or treadmill at home by watching VHS or DVD movies, but only in a certain way.

Choose an action film, and keep it playing for as long as you keep up the exercise, then turn it off the minute you stop. This method has several advantages: First, action films, like dance music, tend to activate the body physiologically, and thus make you want to move. Second, a good film has a hypnotic effect that helps you forget the passage of time. The 20 minutes of prescribed exercise go by faster than they would if your eyes were glued to the clock. Finally, since watching the film after you stop is not allowed, suspense motivates you to begin again the next day, if only to find out what happens. (Machines make noise and exercise tends to disrupt concentration, so it's wise to avoid psychological drama that relies heavily on subtleties of dialogue. Furthermore, as laughter is not compatible with physical exercise, it is also better to avoid comedies.) Get your blood pumping with some action, on the screen and off.

Turning to Others

Up to now, we have talked only about approaches to the emotional brain that center on the individual. Cardiac coherence, EMDR, dawn simulation, acupuncture, nutrition, and exercise all focus on the individual and his or her body. However, the role of the emotional brain is not simply to govern the inner physiology of the body. Its other function is equally important: to regulate the balance of our emotional connections and to ensure that we always have our place in the pack, the group, the tribe, and the family. Anxiety and depression are often the signals of distress that our emotional brain sends out when it detects a threat to the equilibrium in our social relations. To pacify and live in harmony with the emotional brain, we need to govern our relations with others more gracefully. In fact, what we need are a few principles of emotional hygiene. These principles are as simple and effective as they are generally ignored by most of us.

1 1

Love Is a Biological Need

Michelle's mother hands back her report card. "How can you be so dumb? You'll never amount to anything. Good thing I've got your sister!"

Jack's wife breaks a plate on the rim of the kitchen sink. "Are you finally going to listen to me? I'm fed up with screaming at you! How can anybody be so self-centered?"

A few days after starting his job, Edgar looks for some information in another department of his new company. A colleague he hasn't yet met comes up and says, "I don't know who you are, but you don't belong here, so get the hell out!"

For the third time this week, Sophia's neighbors are partying till two in the morning. In retaliation, she takes out her garbage pails at 7 A.M., making as much noise as she can. "That'll teach them," she mutters.

Nothing makes our emotional brain wince more than conflicts with the people who surround us. Whether we like it or not, even conflicts with our neighbors—who are, after all, "outsiders"—can leave a lingering pocket of resentment and anger in our day.

On the other hand, our heart melts at the sight of a smiling child taking her father's hand, looking him in the eye and saying, "I love you, Daddy." Or of an elderly woman on her deathbed looking at her husband and telling him, "I've been very happy with you. I have no regrets. I can leave in peace. And when you feel the breeze on your face, you'll know it's me cuddling you." Or at the sight of a refugee hugging a doctor from a relief group and saying again, "You've been sent by God. I was so frightened, and you've saved my daughter!"

In both positive and negative cases, we react to the emotional connection between people. When people are "emotionally violent" with each other—when they treat each other in cruel and aggressive ways—we all suffer, even when we are mere witnesses. When instead, they say what they are feeling ("I love you," "I've been happy," "I was frightened") and use this feeling to get closer and touch each other's hearts, rather than retaliate or punish, we cannot help but be moved.

Movie directors and advertising executives have expert insight into what gets a reaction out of us. They try to persuade us to buy a particular brand of coffee, for example, by implying that its aroma brings people—friends, couples, a mother and daughter—closer. These marketing messages can be appealing on such an elemental level that depressed people frequently confess that tears come to their eyes during some TV commercials. Usually, they don't know why, but often it's simply because they have just witnessed a show of affection between two people. This feeling of connection, of intimacy, is precisely what they long for most in their own lives.

Over the last 30 years, rates of depression have been steadily increasing in Western societies. In the last 10 years, consumption of antidepressants has doubled in the most advanced Western countries.[1] Today, more than 11 million Americans are taking antidepressants.[2] These data are so stark that most of us and our institutions prefer not to think about them. We all go along in blissful denial and stock up on Prozac. We tell ourselves that someday this will all get resolved. But things are not getting resolved. They are getting worse. If someone asked me where to begin to reverse this trend, I would reply that we need to start by confronting the violence in daily relationships, in couples, with our children, or our neighbors, and in the workplace.[3] We need to become more respectful of the needs of our emotional brain for harmony and connectedness. There is no way around what evolution has wired us to want and feel in relationships.

The Physiology of Love

One part of the emotional brain distinguishes mammals from reptiles. From the standpoint of evolution, the basic difference is that baby mammals are vulnerable. These fragile youngsters are incapable of surviving for several days, weeks, or years without constant attention from their parents.

Human beings represent the most extreme example. Nurturing our infants requires the longest parental investment of all creatures. In human beings, like other mammals, evolution has thus created limbic structures in the brain that make us particularly sensitive to our children's needs.* Evolution has wired our brain with the instinct to respond to them—nourishing our children, keeping them warm, cuddling them, protecting them, teaching them how to hunt, to gather, and to defend themselves. Our brain has been designed to secure a relationship that is indispensable to the survival of the species. It is the foundation of our profound capacity to form social relations with others—in a pack, a tribe, or a family.

---

*Even though they are oviparous, birds have some of the same limbic structures as mammals. This is probably because at birth their young are similarly helpless and dependent on the care of parents.

A specific region in our emotional brain is even responsible for the cries of distress we let out—as babies—when we are separated from those to whom we are attached.[4] That same region is also responsible for our instinctive reaction to these cries. Already at birth, the baby's emotional brain calls out to his mother: "Are you there?" and again and again, the mother's emotional brain is compelled to answer him, "Yes, I'm here!" These cries and our instinctive reply to them make the "reflex circuit" of relationships between beings—animals or humans. This circuit is the foundation for all vocal communication—for bird songs, lowing, roaring, hooting, barking, meowing, squealing, for all poetry, and for songs. The remarkable tug of music on our hearts—especially the human voice singing—probably has its roots here. Music acts directly on the emotional brain, a lot more effectively than language or mathematics.

This limbic communication does not exist in reptiles—so much the better for them, in a way. If baby lizards, crocodiles, or snakes let their parents know where they were, they would be quickly eaten up. The same is true for sharks. In contrast, mother dolphins or whales constantly use sound to communicate with their offspring, and these marine mammals sing in ways that scientists unhesitatingly compare to human communication. In fact, we humans can experience loving relationships with virtually all mammals and with a good many birds (parrots and parakeets are remarkably affectionate domestic animals). But neither boas nor iguanas will respond with affection to the love you may feel for them.

The emotional brain is thus made to send out and receive messages on the channel of affect, the outward expression of our emotions. Such communication turns out to play a key role in the organism's survival, and not just in procuring food and warmth. We now know that emotional contact is a real *biological need* for mammals, on a par with food and oxygen. Modern biological science has rediscovered this, despite itself.

Hardwired for Touch

In the eighties, progress in intensive care enabled premature infants to survive at an earlier and earlier age. In hermetically closed incubators equipped with ultraviolet light, conditions can be artificially regulated with enough precision to sustain life in these tiny human bodies. So small are these babies that interns call them, affectionately, "the little shrimps."

But the frail nervous systems of these babies had trouble withstanding the handling required by their care, so specialists devised ways of caring for them without physical contact. Signs on incubators read: "DO NOT TOUCH."

The cries of distress emerging from these incubators, despite their soundproofing, were heartrending, even to the most hardened nurses. But they conscientiously ignored the cries and went about their important healing work. Nevertheless, despite the ideal conditions of temperature, humidity, and oxygen, the food meticulously measured down to the last milligram, and the soothing ultraviolet light, the infants did not grow. Scientifically, their stunted growth was a mystery, almost a slap in the face. Under such perfect conditions, how could nature refuse to cooperate?

Doctors and researchers shook their heads—what more could they do? They consoled themselves with the observation that once the infants—those who survived—were out of the incubator, their weight quickly caught up.

But one day in a neonatal department, the doctors observed that some babies seemed to be growing normally while still in their incubators. Yet nothing had changed in their treatment protocols—almost nothing.

To the doctors' great surprise, an investigation revealed that the infants who were growing were being looked after by the same night nurse, a woman who had just begun to work in the department.

When she was questioned, the young woman was reticent at first—she didn't want to draw fire—but ended up confessing. Turns out, she was incapable of resisting the cries of her tiny patients. With misgivings at first, because it was forbidden, but with growing confidence, she had begun several weeks earlier to rub each baby's back to calm their cries. As none of the dire effects foreseen had actually come about, and because the babies did indeed seem to calm down, she had continued—secretly, of course.

Since then, at Duke University, Professor Saul Schonberg, M.D., Ph.D., and his team have confirmed this outcome in a series of experiments with rat pups isolated at birth. Their research has found that without physical contact, every cell in the tiny animal's organism literally refuses to develop. In all of the rat pup's cells, the part of the genome producing the enzymes needed for growth no longer expresses itself; in effect, the whole body enters a state similar to hibernation. However, if a damp brush gently strokes a baby rat's back—like a mother rat licking her pup in response to its cries—the enzyme production immediately starts up again—and so does the pup's growth. Emotional contact is undeniably necessary to growth and even to survival.[5]

In the first modern orphanages around the middle of the 20th century, nurses received orders not to touch children or even play with them, for fear of contracting and spreading contagious diseases. Despite the excellent physical care and nourishment they received, 40 percent of the orphans who came down with measles died. Outside of these "hygienic" orphanages, fewer than 1 *child in 100*—less than 1 percent!—died from that generally mild disease.[6]

In 1981, David Hubel, M.D., and Torsten Wiesel, M.D., two Harvard researchers, received the Nobel Prize in Medicine for their fundamental investigation into the way the visual system develops. Among their discoveries was the demonstration that the visual cortex develops normally only if it gets adequate stimulation during a critical period at the very beginning of life.[7] Today we are discovering that this is also true for the emotional brain.

Experience in several dreadful Romanian orphanages, where even recently children were being attached to their bed and fed like animals, confirmed this need. Observations of their plight have shown what happens to small members of our species when they do not receive emotional nourishment—the majority die. Since then, researchers in Detroit, at Wayne State University, have demonstrated that the emotional brain in young survivors of Romanian orphanages is often atrophied—perhaps irreversibly.[8]

By chance, Myron Hofer, M.D., Ph.D., of Cornell University, discovered how damage to emotional relationships in mammals disorganizes their physiology. He was studying the physiology of rat pups, when one morning he noticed that one of the mother rats had left her cage during the night. The abandoned offspring had a heart rhythm 50 percent below normal. Hofer first thought this rhythm was due to lack of heat. To check his hypothesis, he covered a small electric heater with a sock and placed it in the midst of the tiny, hairless rats. To his great surprise, nothing changed. From experiment to experiment, Hofer was able to show that not only cardiac rhythm, but 15 other physiological functions depended on the presence of the mother rat—in fact, on her demonstrations of maternal caring. Chief among these functions are the regulation of periods of sleep and nocturnal waking, blood pressure, body temperature, and even the activity of immune cells like lymphocytes B and T—their defense against infection (see "Mother Love and the Physiology of the Newborn," on page 168).[9] In the end, he came to this astonishing conclusion: The principal source of the baby rats' biological regulation was . . . mother love.

In human beings, research has established that the quality of the relationship between parents and child—defined by the parents' empathy and their response to the child's emotional needs—will determine the balance of the child's parasympathetic system some years

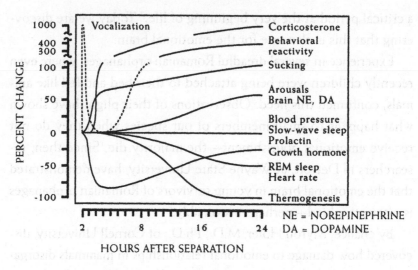

NE = NOREPINEPHRINE
DA = DOPAMINE

HOURS AFTER SEPARATION

MOTHER LOVE AND THE PHYSIOLOGY OF THE NEWBORN

In the hours following separation from its mother, the baby rat's physiology becomes literally unglued. In a "normal" state, its different physical functions are aligned on each other, within specific ranges. After separation, everything is disrupted, as if the newborn baby's close-knit physiology had come apart. (M. A. Hofer, "Early Social Relationships: A Psychologist View," Child Development, Vol. 58. Illustration by Hofer.)

later. And the parasympathetic system is the precise factor that promotes cardiac coherence and resistance to stress and depression.[10]

"Does Your Wife Show You Her Love?"

We now know that in all mammals, including human beings, the physiological balance of babies depends on the love they receive. Is it really surprising that this is also true for adults?

A study in the *British Medical Journal* has shown that the average survival time of elderly widowers is far shorter than that of men of the same age whose wife is still alive.[11] Another study demonstrates that men with cardiovascular disease who said "yes" to the question "Does your wife show you her love?" had half as many symptoms as the others. And the more risk factors (cholesterol, high blood pressure, stress) these men accumulate, the more their wife's love protects them.[12] The reverse phenomenon was shown when 8,500 healthy men were tracked for 5 years. Those who, at the beginning of the survey, recognized themselves in the statement, "My wife doesn't love me," developed three times more ulcers than the others. According to this research, it is better to be a smoker, to suffer from high blood pressure, or to undergo ongoing stress than to not be loved by your wife.[13]

The benefits of emotional support are just as great in women. Out of 1,000 women diagnosed with breast cancer, twice as many who had said they lacked affection died within 5 years.[14] Even among healthy women, those who often feel "despised" by their husbands have more colds, cystitis, and intestinal problems than those whose marital life is harmonious.[15] Women who live together, or even merely share an office, often have synchronized menstrual cycles,[16] but the phenomenon is stronger when there is a real emotional connection between them—when they are friends, rather than just roommates or colleagues.

The lesson from all of this research is simple. The physiology of social mammals is not separate from the rest. At all times, its optimum functioning depends on our relations with others, especially with those with whom we are close emotionally. In *A General Theory of Love*, a wonderful book on the emotional brain and its workings, three psychiatrists from the University of San Francisco, Tom Lewis, M.D., Fari Amini, M.D., and Richard Lannon, M.D., have named this phenomenon "limbic regulation." In their words, "A relationship *is* a physiological process, as real and as potent as any pill or surgical procedure."[17] But obviously, this is an idea that still has trouble getting accepted—even though it is fully validated by science—perhaps because the human connection cannot be patented, and therefore does not contribute to the sale of medicines.

Animals Can Heal Us, Too

At the hospital where I practiced in Pittsburgh, other physicians often asked my advice before discharging a depressed elderly patient after bypass surgery or hospitalization for a fractured hip. Usually, I was the last person they consulted. The colleagues preceding me had already prescribed a long list of medicines: antiarrhythmic, antihypertensive, anti-inflammatory, antacid. They expected me to carry the ball and add my own "anti" to the list—an antidepressant or anxiolytic (anti-anxiety medication).

Often, however, the cause of depression was clear. The old man or woman had been living alone for years, and was no longer going out very much because of frail health. No longer playing bingo with friends. No longer being visited by their children or grandchildren, who had left for California, Boston, or New York. These men and women were idling away the hours in front of television screens. Would these patients honestly feel like looking after themselves? Even if antidepressants could have done them good, would they have taken them every day? Probably no more than those other pills, already so hard to distinguish from each other and to take as prescribed.

I really did not feel like adding my two-cents' worth to that confusion. Medicines are not "limbic regulators." So, summoning up all my courage, I would add my recommendation to the patient's medical record: "As far as her depression is concerned, the best thing for this patient would be to get a dog (a small one, obviously, to minimize the risk of a fall). If the patient considers that would be too much work, a cat would do, since it does not need to be taken out. And if a cat still seems too much, a bird or a fish. Finally, if the patient still refuses, then a houseplant."

At the beginning of this campaign, I received slightly irritated calls from the residents in orthopedic or cardiovascular surgery: "We asked you to recommend an antidepressant, not a zoo. What are we going to write on the discharge prescription? There aren't any household pets at the pharmacy."

However I answered, my explanations seemed convincing only to myself. My colleagues invariably ended up prescribing an antidepressant themselves, mumbling about how useless psychiatrists really were. They were undoubtedly convinced that they were defending the cause of modern scientific medicine against the ever-threatening, obscuring specter of "old-wives' remedies."

I soon realized that my approach was not working and that I was doing damage to my reputation as chief of the psychiatry division of the hospital. Instead of backing down, I prepared a document summing up various scientific studies on the question. From that point on, I attached the document to my recommendations in the patient's record.

I hoped to inform my colleagues of certain remarkable results with which they didn't seem to be familiar, such as one study from the *American Journal of Cardiology* about men and women whose infarctions had been accompanied by dangerous arrhythmias. The patients were tracked for more than a year, and those who had had a household pet faced only one-sixth the likelihood of dying during the year compared to all the others.[18] Or yet another study, in which older people with household pets had much better psychological resistance to life's difficulties and went a lot less often to the doctor's.[19] I also called their attention to a study from a group at Harvard showing that simply looking after a plant lowered the mortality rate of residents in a retirement home by 50 percent.[20] I cited research on AIDS patients showing that cat or dog owners were better protected from depression.[21] Finally, I referred to the font of all knowledge in my colleagues' eyes— the *Journal of the American Medical Association*. In 1996, it published a study about handicapped people who were virtually unable to move around unaided, very similar to the elderly patients I had been asked to see. This study showed that these people were happier and had greater self-esteem and a distinctly larger network of friends and relations if they had the companionship of a dog.[22] In fact, another study found that the mere presence of an animal by your side makes you "more attractive" to others.[23]

Even stockbrokers feel better if they have a household pet. With one of the most stressful professions imaginable, they are constant victims of market ups and downs over which they have no control, yet they still have to meet their sales targets. It is hardly surprising that a good many of them suffer early from high blood pressure. Karen Allen, Ph.D., from the University of Buffalo, conducted an unconventional study on a group of brokers in her city. Antihypertensive medications brought their blood pressure down below the initial alarming average of 160/100. However, in moments of stress, they still showed sudden peaks of blood pressure above those numbers.

To a randomly selected half of the stockbrokers, Dr. Allen allocated either a dog or a cat. (They had the opportunity to choose one or the other.) Six months later, the results spoke for themselves: Those who had received household pets were no longer reacting to stress in the same way. Not only had their blood pressure stabilized, even in periods of stress, but their performance on stress-inducing tasks—such as rapid mental arithmetic and public speaking—was significantly better. They made fewer mistakes, suggesting that they had more control over their emotions and thus over their concentration.[24] In another study, Dr. Allen was able to show that older women (over 70) who lived alone but with pets had the same blood pressure as women of 25 with active social lives.[25]

My "enclosure" turned out to be effective. After that, nobody ever made the slightest comment. I no longer heard interns snicker behind my back when I left one of my "zoological" recommendations in their patient's file. On the other hand, alas, I do not think that a single patient ever went home with a cat or *without* his or her prescription for Prozac.

The idea that a loving relationship is *in itself* a physiological remedy, comparable to taking medication, rests on sound scientific ground— but it simply has not yet taken hold in the medical establishment.

The Pets of Sarajevo

Owners of a household pet do not need anyone to prove scientifically what they experience in their everyday life, even if those circumstances become extraordinary.[26] In 1993, Sarajevo was under bombardment and constant threat from snipers. Except for a few "humanitarian" rations, there had been almost nothing to eat for almost a year. All the shops had been looted. None of the windows was still intact. The city parks had been turned into cemeteries and were running out of space. It was no longer safe to venture out in the street for fear of a stray bullet or a sniper shot.

Yet in that exhausted and agonizing city, where anything stirring came from the clash of arms, you could still see men, women, and children walking their dogs. "You have to take him out," said a man in the street, "and then you forget the war for a moment. When you devote your time to something else, you forget a little."

In the only undamaged room left in their apartment, an old couple had kept a dog and a cat they had found wounded in the street at the beginning of the siege. They thought that after a few weeks, when the animals were better, they would let them go. A year later, they were still there.

Nadja and Thomaslov shared whatever meager rations they managed to get from time to time with the animals. The cat preferred the powdered milk from the French relief package. "He's an aristocrat," they laughingly said. But when he was really hungry, he would take the American rations, which were a little easier to obtain.

The dog had seven puppies in front of the building, and five of them survived because the residents brought them leftovers whenever they could. "We are taking care of them because we feel that we need something to live around us," Nadja said. "We are feeding the birds, too, because we need them around us. We are not evil. This thing reminds us of peace, you know? Everyday peace and what we used to have. We have to believe that we are going to survive."

That was Sarajevo in 1993. In the midst of a nightmare, when there is nothing left, there is still love, even for a dog. To still be able to give something, to feel human, to feel that you are still useful to someone, is a drive stronger than hunger, stronger than fear. When these relationships are disturbed, our physiology is damaged. We experience it as pain. The suffering is emotional, but it is still pain and often more intense, actually, than physical suffering.

Thankfully, this important key to our emotional brain does not depend on a partner's love alone. Actually, it depends on the quality of all our emotional bonds—with our children, our parents, our brothers and sisters, our friends, our animals. What is important is the feeling of being fully oneself with someone else. To be able to show we are weak and vulnerable, as well as strong and radiant. To be able to laugh, but also to cry. To feel that our emotions are understood. To know that we are useful and important to someone. And to have a minimum of warm physical contacts. Quite simply, to be loved.

Like all the plants that turn toward sunlight, we need the light of love and friendship. Without it, we sink into anxiety and depression. Alas, in our society, centrifugal forces are constantly at work to separate us from each other. And when they are not driving us apart, they often lead us to live with verbal violence rather than with love. To govern our physiology for the best, we have to learn to govern our relations with others for the best. And that can be done only if we go to the trouble of learning the foundations of what might be called "emotional communication," only if we decide to learn how to get the most out of our connections with other people. This is the topic of the next three chapters.

12

Enhancing Emotional Communication

> *"Those who find the right words never offend anyone. Yet they speak the truth. Their words are clear but never harsh. They do not take offense, and they do not give it."*
>
> —THE BUDDHA

I had a wonderful friend in Pittsburgh whose family situation was almost a parable. In the family were about 30 cousins, and one of the favorite subjects of conversation at large family reunions was their "terrible" Aunt Esther.

At 85, she continued to inspire a certain terror—now mixed with pity—in her sisters, their children, and even their grandchildren. She had always been cantankerous and difficult. But she had a lively intelligence and had inherited a large fortune from her husband 20 years earlier, and thanks to these two attributes, she often succeeded in imposing her views in family matters. She was continually calling everybody to get news of the family or to ask for help; insisting on somebody chauffeuring her all over the place; complaining that they did not come and see her often enough; and when she felt like it, inviting herself to dinner or even for the weekend. It was obvious that Esther sought affection and gratitude. But her aggressive manner drove away all the people she tried to get closer to.

The 30 cousins were divided into three distinct categories in their relations with their aunt. By far the largest number were those who never said "no" to Aunt Esther directly. They always found an excuse or other to avoid her. Yet, when they had their backs to the wall after all her insistence and arguments, they ended up saying "yes." They did so regretfully so as to avoid her diatribes, her interminable phone calls, and her recriminations. On the other hand, they never called her back, even when they had promised to. They forgot their dates with her, or else they arrived late. Behind her back, they made fun of her. They even tried to wheedle money out of her, sometimes dishonestly. They seemed to think her difficult personality and everything they had to do for her against their will gave them the right to treat her this way.

This type of behavior is called "passive" or "passive aggressive." In traditional societies, it is the most common human reaction when facing an individual in a position of authority who is disliked. Strangely, it is also the most common in modern families and corporations.[1] This is often the behavior of people who see themselves as "sensitive," "respectful of others," "not wanting to make waves," or "preferring to give rather than receive." This behavior did not work much better in George's family than it does in traditional societies or companies. On one hand, these cousins felt "used" by Esther and they felt resentful of her. On the other, Esther, who was very aware of their ill will and suspected their dishonesty, despised them. Moreover, as she had connections in high places and influence among certain decision makers in the city, they often felt her wrath manifested in complications in other parts of their lives.

Fewer cousins found themselves in the second group. One night, Esther had woken one of the cousins up at midnight. Larry, who was not afraid of her, told her that he had had enough of her obnoxious manners. Then, carried away by years of accumulated irritation, he had told her off.

Esther was deeply wounded. But, as she was never at a loss for words, she answered back with two or three comments that wounded him just as much. Larry was never sorry for speaking his mind, but he knew that from that moment on Esther would use the slightest pretext to side against him. And, indeed, in the following years, she never missed an occasion to make her hostility felt, as she did with other family members who had acted the same way with her. Due to Esther's influential friends, Larry's law firm even lost several clients.

True, Aunt Esther no longer pestered Larry and even did her best to avoid him. At least he did not have to deal with her directly anymore. Also, he had had the satisfaction of having stood up to her, after all those years of keeping his feelings inside.

Larry and the other cousins who reacted like him had displayed what is known as "aggressive" behavior. This behavior is less common than the first type and is typically more masculine. But it is not any more effective at solving problems and it usually leads to substantial damage in the end, such as divorce or dismissal from jobs, among other unpleasant side effects. Besides, this type of behavior has been recognized by internists and cardiologists as an important cause of high blood pressure and cardiovascular diseases.[2]

Then there was my friend George, who comprised the third group. George was fully aware of Esther's shortcomings. Still, he not only saw her regularly, but these visits did not seem to burden him. He seemed to have genuine affection for her, and it was reciprocal. In fact, Esther often did him favors, looking after his children, or taking his car to the garage. She had even lent him the money to build an addition to his house and had given him competent advice on redecorating his office.

I knew George because he worked in the same hospital as I did. I always admired how skillfully he handled his relations with his colleagues and subordinates. I marveled, too, at his way of dealing with those inevitable moments of tension that had come up in the course of our friendship of several years.

It took me a long time to grasp what made him different from his other cousins, something that unquestionably enabled him to maintain a valued relationship with someone as difficult as his Aunt Esther. In fact, George was a master of the third kind of behavior, the kind that is neither passive nor aggressive. On his own, he had discovered the principles of good emotional communication—what is sometimes called "nonviolent assertive communication." This is the only communication that enables us to give and receive what we need while remaining respectful of our own limits and the needs of others.

One evening, he invited me to his house for dinner, and I had the opportunity of observing him in action as he dealt with his Aunt Esther. Esther was to accompany him on a trip he was making for the university to a city where she had a lot of connections. That evening, she called George for the third time in two days. She wanted to add several other people to his already full schedule of appointments.

George had had a long day at the hospital. It was late. I knew how much he appreciated dining in peace, especially when he had invited a friend to join him. I wondered how he was going to handle the situation. First, he took a deep breath, then he moved in:

"Esther, you know how much this trip we are taking together means to me and how grateful I am for everything you have done for me." It was true: I knew that he didn't have to force himself to say that. I don't know what Esther said to him, but I felt right away that the tension at the other end of the line had decreased.

Then he went on: "But when you call me three times to say the same thing, after we've already talked for an hour and agreed on these matters, I feel frustrated. I need to feel that we are a team and that you respect my needs just as I respect yours. Can we agree now that we won't go back over the decisions we've already made?"

In 2 minutes, the conversation was over, and he could concentrate on dinner. And he was perfectly serene, as if he had just simply been told his flight schedule. I thought of all the patients over the years who had called me on my beeper at unreasonable hours. If only I had known how to talk to them like that. Only much later did I discover the logic and the well-greased mechanism underneath the quiet strength of my friend George.

The Love Lab of Seattle

At the University of Washington in Seattle, in a place called the "Love Lab," married couples agree to be examined under the microscope of emotions of psychologist John Gottman, Ph.D. While a couple interacts, video cameras pick up the slightest grimace that crosses their faces, even if it lasts only a few tenths of a second. Sensors record variations in their cardiac rhythm and blood pressure. Since Dr. Gottman, author of *The Relationship Cure*, started his Love Lab, more than 100 couples have agreed to talk about their subjects of chronic conflict—the distribution of household tasks, decisions about the children, the management of family finances, relations with in-laws, disagreements over smoking and drinking, and so on.

Dr. Gottman's first discovery is that there are no happy couples—in fact, there are no lasting emotional relationships—without chronic conflict. To the contrary: Couples that have no chronic subjects of dispute should be worried. The absence of conflict is a sign of an emotional distance so great as to preclude an authentic relationship. The second—astonishing—discovery is that Dr. Gottman can analyze a mere 5 minutes—5 minutes!—of an argument between a husband and wife and predict with more than 90 percent accuracy who will remain married and who will divorce within a few years—even if the couple is still in the midst of their honeymoon.[3]

Nothing afflicts our emotional brain and our physiology more than feeling emotionally cut off from those to whom we are most attached—our spouse, our children, our parents. In the Love Lab, a harsh word, or a tiny facial contortion of contempt or disgust—hardly visible to an observer—is enough to speed up the heartbeat in the person to whom the comment is targeted. After a well-aimed jab combined with a bit of disdain, the heart rate will suddenly climb to more than 110.*[4]

Once the emotional brain is aroused in this way, it turns off the cognitive brain's ability to reason rationally. As we have seen, the prefrontal cortex is "off-line." Men, in particular, are very sensitive to what Dr. Gottman calls "emotional flooding." Once their physiology is aroused, they are "flooded" by their emotions and they think only in terms of defense and attack. They no longer look for responses that will restore calm to the situation. Many women also react the same way. When we hear this exchange—from one of Dr. Gottman's studies—it sounds terribly familiar:

Fred: Did you pick up my dry cleaning?

Ingrid (in a mocking tone): "Did you pick up my dry cleaning?" Pick up your own damn dry cleaning. What am I, your maid?

Fred: Hardly. If you were a maid, at least you'd know how to clean.[5]

During that exchange, Fred's and Ingrid's physiology quickly becomes disorganized (I imagine that their heart rate variability would also be very chaotic, though this was not measured in the Love Lab). The effects on the relationship are disastrous.

With compelling arguments, Gottman defines this type of negative situation as featuring the "four horsemen of the apocalypse," four

---

*For men the normal heart rate is usually about 70 beats per minute; for women, approximately 80.

attitudes that wreak havoc in all the relationships that they encounter on their passage. These conveyed attitudes activate the
emotional brain of the other person to such an extent that the other
party can only respond with meanness or else withdraw like a
wounded animal. If we rely on the four horsemen for communication, we are literally assured of not getting what we desire out of the
relationship, yet we almost always call these warriors up to the front
of our emotional battles.

1. **Criticism.** The first horseman is *criticism*, criticizing someone's
character instead of simply stating a grievance. An example of a criticism: "You're late again. You only think of yourself." A grievance
would be: "It's nine o'clock. You said you would be here at eight. It's
the second time this week. I'm lonely and upset when I wait for you
like this."

Criticism: "I'm fed up with picking up your clothes. Your messiness is exasperating!" Grievance: "When you leave your things all
over the kitchen, it bothers me. In the morning when I'm having my
coffee, I need order around me to feel good. Could you try to pick
up at night before you go to bed?"

Dr. Gottman gives an infallible recipe for changing a legitimate
grievance with a good chance of being heard into a criticism certain to spark resentment, ill will, and a virulent counterattack. All
you need to do is tack on a scornful, "What's wrong with you?"

What is so surprising about these observations is how obvious
they are. We all know exactly how we *don't* like to be treated. It is
hard for us, on the other hand, to say exactly how we *would* like to be
treated. Yet, our gratitude immediately overflows when someone addresses us in an emotionally intelligent manner.

I remember an unexpected lesson I received one day over the
telephone. I had been waiting over 20 minutes while an airline
ticket agent looked into the status of my reservation. The flight
was for that same afternoon, and I was impatient and worried.

When she finally admitted that she could not find my reservation, I burst out, "What!? But that's crazy. What use are you if you can't find a reservation?"

As I was speaking these words, I was already sorry. I knew very well that I was alienating the person I most needed to solve my problem. But I did not know how to get out of this jam. I thought it would be ridiculous to apologize. (In fact, it is never too early or too late to apologize, but that was something I had not yet learned.) To my great surprise, she was the one who saved me: "When you raise your voice, sir, I can't concentrate on helping you."

I was lucky; she had just given me the perfect opportunity to apologize without losing face. I did so immediately. A few moments later, we were once again talking like two adults trying to solve a problem. When I explained how much the trip mattered to me, she even changed into a real ally; she broke a rule by giving me a seat on a flight that was theoretically blocked.

I was the psychiatrist, but she was the one who had completely mastered the emotions of the conversation. That evening, I imagined her on her way home, undoubtedly more relaxed than I was. That experience led me to learn about nonviolent emotional communication. In fact, in my years of training, nobody had considered it important or useful to teach it to me.

2. Contempt. Dr. Gottman's second horseman, the most violent and dangerous for our limbic balance, is *contempt*. Contempt shows its face in insults, of course. From the mildest—some would say underhanded—such as "your behavior is inappropriate," to the most conventional and violent like "poor thing, you really are dumb," or the common "you're a jerk," or the simple but no less deadly "you're ridiculous."

Sarcasm can also be very hurtful. Listen again to Fred's response to Ingrid: "If you were a maid, at least you'd know how to clean."

Sarcasm can sometimes be funny at the movies (and even there, it all depends). But it is not funny at all in a real relationship. Yet, in an attempt to be clever or witty—often at the expense of others—sarcasm is precisely the tool to which we often turn, sometimes with relish. I know a major French journalist with a very sharp wit who spent more than 15 years in what she considers to be a very successful course of psychoanalysis. One day, long after her analysis was over, we were talking about ways of dealing with conflict. She told me, "When I feel attacked, I try to destroy my adversary. If I manage to smash him to smithereens, I'm happy."

Facial expressions are often all it takes to communicate contempt: eyes rolling toward the ceiling in response to what has just been said, the corners of the mouth turned down with eyes narrowing in reaction to the other person. When the disparager who sends us these signals is someone we live or work with, they go straight to the heart. And that makes a peaceful resolution of the situation practically impossible. How can we reason or speak peaceably when the message we receive is that we inspire disdain?

3. **Counterattack** and 4. **Stonewalling.** The third and fourth horsemen are *counterattack* and *stonewalling.* When we are attacked, the two responses the emotional brain offers us are fight and flight (these are the famous alternatives described by the great American physiologist, Walter B. Cannon, in a classical description in 1929). These responses have been engraved in our genes over millions of years of evolution, and they are, indeed, the most effective choices for insects or reptiles.

Now, in all conflicts, the problem of counterattack is that it leads, in turn, to only two possible outcomes. In the worst of cases, it provokes an escalation of violence. Wounded by my counterattack, the other person will raise the stakes. This horseman is very active in the Middle East, of course, but also in all the kitchens of the world where couples clash. Escalation usually carries on until there is a permanent physical separation between the warring factions—the destruction of the relationship by dismissal, divorce . . . or murder.

In the best of cases, the counterattack "succeeds" and the other party is defeated by our verve. Or victory is obtained—as parents often do with their children, and men sometimes do with women—with a slap. The law of the jungle has spoken and the reptile in us is satisfied. But that kind of victory inevitably leaves the vanquished wounded and sore, and this wound only widens the emotional gap and only makes living together more difficult. A violent counterattack has never inspired an opponent to beg forgiveness and take the aggressor in her arms. Yet, even in torn relationships this outcome is precisely what we are yearning for.

The other option—stonewalling—is a masculine specialty that's particularly upsetting to women. Stonewalling often foreshadows the final phase of a disintegrating relationship, be it a marriage or a professional association.

After weeks or months of criticism, of attacks and counterattacks, one of the protagonists will choose "flight," and abandon the battlefield, at least emotionally. While the other person still seeks contact and offers to talk, the second party scowls, looks at his feet, or hides behind his newspaper, "waiting for the storm to blow over." The antagonist, exasperated by this tactic that supposes to ignore her completely, talks louder and louder and eventually starts shouting.

Stonewalling is the stage of the flying plate or—when the person who turns into a "brick wall" is a woman—of possibly getting beaten up. Physical violence is a desperate attempt to reconnect with the other who has left the scene, to try to make her hear what we are experiencing emotionally, to make her feel our pain. Obviously, it never succeeds. In *The Hunchback of Notre-Dame*, Victor Hugo magnificently illustrated this vain and violent pursuit of the love object who ignores you. To feel recognized by Esmeralda, who persisted in ignoring him and rejecting his advances, Abbé Frollo ended up torturing her and sending her to her death.

Emotional withdrawal is not an effective way to deal with conflicts. As Dr. Gottman has shown in the lab, and Hugo described before him, stonewalling often leads to a sorry end.

Saying It All while Doing No Harm

Thanks to the Seattle Love Lab, we now understand, to an unprecedented extent, what is going on in the heads and hearts of people in conflict, and how they often head straight into a wall. Naturally, we have every reason to believe that the same reflexes and same mistakes undermine the course of conflicts outside of marriages as well.

These conflicts may involve our children, our parents, our in-laws, or, most often, our boss and our colleagues in the office. But what, then, are the principles of effective communication? Communication that gets the message across without alienating the person who receives it? Communication that, to the contrary, invites respect and makes that person want to help us?

One of the masters of effective emotional communication is the psychologist Marshall Rosenberg, Ph.D., author of the book *Nonviolent Communication*. Born in a poor and violent neighborhood of Detroit, he was very young when he became passionately interested in intelligent ways to solve conflict without violence. He has taught and practiced in many circumstances and parts of the world where conflict management is indispensable. These include schools in difficult neighborhoods and major firms undergoing reorganization, everywhere from the Middle East to South Africa.[6]

The first principle of nonviolent communication is to replace judgment—that is, criticism—by an objective statement of facts. Saying, "You are doing a poor job," or even "This report isn't good," immediately puts the other person on the defensive. Being simply objective and specific is much better: "In this report, there are three ideas needed in order to communicate our message that seem to be missing."

The more specific and objective we are, the more likely the other person will be to react to our words as a legitimate attempt to communicate rather than as an attack on his or her being. Rosenberg cites a study that examined the relationship between a country's literature and the violence of its citizens. According to this research, the more often literary works of the country contain statements labeling people as "good" or "bad," the more frequently acts of violence are registered in the justice system.[7]

The second principle is to avoid any judgment of the other while concentrating entirely on what we feel. This reservation of judgment is the master key to emotional communication. If I talk about what I feel, nobody can argue with me. For example, if I say, "You never think about me; it's your usual self-centeredness," the person I am talking to can only challenge what I have said. If, on the other hand, I say, "Today was my birthday and you didn't remember it. When you do that, I feel lonely," the person cannot question my feelings. She may think I should not have them, but that is not for her to decide; they are who I am.

The whole point is to describe the situation with sentences beginning with "I" rather than "you." By talking about myself, and only myself, I am no longer criticizing the other person; I am not attacking either. I am expressing my feelings, and therefore, I am being authentic and open. If I'm skilled and really honest with myself, I can even go so far as to expose my vulnerability by showing how the other person has hurt me. I may be vulnerable because I have exposed one of my weaknesses, but in most cases, it is precisely this honesty that will disarm the adversary. My candor will make the other person want to cooperate—insofar, of course, as that person is invested in our relationship.

This technique is exactly what George was doing with his Aunt Esther ("When you call me . . . I feel frustrated") and also what the ticket agent used with me ("When you raise your voice, I can't concentrate on helping you"). They talked about only two things: what had just taken place—objectively, and therefore beyond judgment—and what feelings they experienced in response. They said not a word about what they thought of their "opponent," because that would have been useless.

According to Dr. Rosenberg, what's even more effective is not only to say what we feel, but also to express the disappointed needs we had. "When you arrive late for a movie date, I feel frustrated because I really like to see the beginning of the film. It's important for me to see the whole show in order to enjoy it." Or, "When you wait a whole week to call me and tell me what you're up to, I'm afraid something has happened. I need to be reassured more often that everything is all right." Or at work, "When you allow a document to circulate with spelling mistakes, I feel personally embarrassed. My image and the image of the whole team is affected. Our reputation is very important to me, especially since we have worked so hard to win respect."

I teach this approach to communication to young doctors who are sorely in need of a method for dealing with difficult patients. I actually give them a step-by-step procedure which they often write down on a card and keep in their pockets, just in case they have to prepare for a difficult encounter.

Dr. Rosenberg talks about a participant in his workshop who told him the following story: This man had started to refer to a card, like the one my students use, to put what he had learned into practice with his children. At the beginning, it was obviously a little embarrassing, sometimes even ridiculous. His children had immediately pointed out how stilted his approach was. But, as a conscientious beginner, he had looked at his card and addressed that very scorn with the procedure he was learning: "When you tell me I'm ridiculous, just as I'm trying to improve our relationship and be a better father to you, you make me sad. I need to feel that it also matters to you that we change the way we've been talking to each other."

His new approach worked; the kids began to listen, and their relationship was improving. He went on in the same vein for several weeks—long enough, in fact, to dispense with the card. Then one day, while he was arguing with his children over television, he lost his temper and forgot about his nonviolent resolutions. His 4-year-old son burst out with some urgency in his voice, "Daddy, go get your card!"

The Six-Point Cue Card for Handling Conflict

The card I use and give to young doctors bears the acronym: "STABEN." These initials sum up the six key points of an effective nonviolent approach. It may offer you your best chances of getting what you want at home, at work, with the police, and even with your car mechanic. These initials stand for:

S for SOURCE. Make sure, to begin with, that you are dealing with the person who is the source of the problem and has the means to solve it. This may sound terribly obvious, but it is usually not our first reaction.

Imagine that, in front of the whole team, a colleague says something disagreeable to me about my work (or my partner, in front of my friends, about my overcooked salmon). It will be completely useless to complain about it later to other colleagues or to my mother over the telephone, yet that is precisely what I will most be tempted to do. If I do, in the best scenario, my disparager will never hear about it. At worst, others will repeat what I said with the usual distortions and exaggerations, and I will look like a whining coward.

To win the respect and change the behavior of my colleague or my partner, I must speak directly to him or her. And I am the only person who can do so. Naturally, facing them is a lot harder and I have no desire to do it. But it is the only approach that stands a chance to improve the relationship. I must go to the source of the problem.

T for TIME and PLACE. Make sure the discussion takes place at a favorable time in a protected, private place. Usually, confronting your aggressor in public or in a corridor is not a good idea, even though your grievance is nonviolent. Nor is it sometimes wise to start the conversation immediately when the wound is still raw or the other party is under stress. A better way would be to choose a place where you can talk in peace and to make sure that the other person is fully available.

A for AMICABLE APPROACH. If you want the other party to hear what you have to say, you first have to make sure that this person is listening. There is no surer way of guaranteeing failure than adopting an aggressive or peremptory tone at the onset. As Dr. Gottman demonstrated in his Love Lab, if one of the protagonists feels attacked, he will tend to be "flooded" by his emotions, even before the conversation gets under way. After that, nothing will help.

Make certain, therefore, that the other person feels at ease from your very first words. Open your antagonist's ears, rather than shut them. Do you know the sweetest sound in the English language? It's the sound of the listener's own name. Psychologists call it the "cocktail party phenomenon." Imagine you are attending a cocktail party, surrounded by a crowd of people conversing. You are, nevertheless, totally absorbed by the conversation you are having with another person. You do not hear anything from the dialogues going on around you, as they are filtered and eliminated by your focused attention.

And then, suddenly, in another group, someone says your name. Immediately you hear it and turn your head. Your name—this one word, more than any other—has the power to attract your attention, just as your name will leap out at you from a page of dense text.

We are more receptive to our name than to any other word. Thus, whatever you intend to say to your disparager, begin by addressing him by his name. Then say something positive, even if it is a stretch, provided that it is true. This positive perspective may sometimes be hard to find, but it is very important. For example, if you intend to complain because your boss criticized you in public, you could say, "David, I appreciate all the opportunities to get feedback from you. That helps me advance in my work." Remember how George began his conversation with Esther: "Esther, you know how much this trip we are making together means to me, and how grateful I am to you."

Beginning on a positive note is not always easy. The first words may even stick a bit in your throat. Still, the effort is worth it. The door to communication is now open.

B for OBJECTIVE BEHAVIOR. Next, you must get to the heart of the matter. Explain the behavior that motivates your grievance, while confining your description to what happened, and nothing more, without the slightest allusion to a moral judgment. You must say, "When you did such and such," and that's it. You must not say, for example, "When you acted like a pervert," but rather, "When you referred to my panties in public."

E for EMOTION. After the description of the facts must come the emotions you experienced as a result of them. Here, you must avoid the trap of talking about your anger, which is often the most obvious emotion. For example, don't say, "When you shouted in front of everybody that my dress was ridiculous (objective behavior), you made me angry." Anger is already an emotion directed toward the other, not the expression of an inner hurt, and it is likely to evoke defensiveness. You'll find it much more powerful and effective to talk about yourself: "I felt hurt," or "The experience was humiliating for me."

   N for NEED. You may stop once you have expressed your true emotion, but it is even more effective to mention your disappointed hopes or the need you feel that has not been recognized: "I need security at work, to know that I won't be humiliated or wounded by caustic remarks, especially from someone as important as you." Or, if your spouse has haughtily ignored you during a dinner party: "I need to feel in contact with you, to feel that I matter to you, even when we are surrounded with friends."

   I know very well that there is something slightly artificial about this procedure, especially when there are so few people around us who can serve as models. You might think, "It would be great if I had the courage to talk like that. But it's impossible. Not with *my* boss," or "Not with *my* husband," "Not with *my* children," "Not with *my* mother-in-law."

   The problem is simple. You have your choice of only three ways to react in a situation of conflict: passivity (or passive-aggression), the most common and least satisfactory reaction; aggression, which is not really any more effective and is a lot more dangerous; or "nonviolent assertiveness"—in other words, nonviolent emotional communication.

   Nevertheless, there are circumstances when it is better to be passive or aggressive than to undertake the more demanding process of assertive communication. An issue may be so trivial, for example, that it does not deserve our time or attention. It is then perfectly legitimate to be "passive" and to accept an insult or to let oneself be manipulated without reacting. I choose this option, for example, when someone honks at me in traffic or when a sales clerk is rude. On the other hand, in emergencies or moments of danger, it is normal to be "aggressive" and to impose orders without any explanation. That is the way the armed forces work, precisely because their whole purpose is to function in the face of immediate danger. Parents do this, too, when they scream at a child who is about to cross the street without paying attention to oncoming traffic.

But whatever the situation, there are only three ways of reacting. In each instance, it is up to us to choose: Will we take on, or give up, the challenge of effective emotional communication? Nothing leads to more stress, anxiety, and depression than unmanaged, unsuccessful relationships with those who matter in our lives. And it is completely up to us, completely in our hands, to change that. The STABEN process is a very solid first step in that direction.

Fortunately, all relationships do not involve conflict. The other aspect of communication, which is generally neglected, is almost as important: knowing how to make the most of opportunities to deepen our relationships with others. One of the simplest ways is to learn how to be fully present when someone is suffering and he or she needs our help. There again, what is important is to find the words so that the current of emotion can pass from one brain to the other, effectively and immediately. This exchange calls for another technique, one that's actually easier to use, probably because it holds fewer risks for us.

13

Listening with the Heart

The first year I was asked to teach physicians at my hospital how to listen to their patients, I remember thinking that I did not have much to offer them. I knew what their most common problem was: the patient who comes to see them about her "headaches" and starts crying in their office. I knew how uncomfortable these young doctors could get when a mother of five children unexpectedly announced in tears that her husband had left her. At that moment, the doctors' overpowering concern centered on how much time this was going to take and how it would affect the overcrowded waiting room. They would say to themselves, "There goes my afternoon schedule!"

To me, as a psychiatrist, it was just the reverse. When a patient broke down in tears, I knew I was on the right track. Because emotion was involved, I knew we were getting to the truth—all we had to do was follow the trail the patient had just opened.

But again, as a psychiatrist, I was in an entirely different situation from my colleagues. Their appointments lasted 10 to 15 minutes; mine were never less than 30 minutes, and usually were an hour or more. The methods of communication I had learned—passive and attentive listening, punctuated with "Hmm . . . hmm . . ." or "Tell me more about your mother"—drew out long effusions. They suited me fine, but they did not fit in with the tight schedules of a surgeon, a cardiologist, or a busy family doctor.

I was scheduled to teach a course, "Managing Difficult Patients," as part of my academic load. I had to find something more useful to teach my colleagues than going "Hmm . . . hmm," and leaning their head to one side. I also wanted it to be something more humane than sending patients home in a hurry with a prescription for Prozac in their pockets. And it was not supposed to take more than 10 minutes.

You never learn more about something than when you have to teach it to somebody else. As I was researching the subject, I discovered the work of Marian R. Stuart, Ph.D., and Joseph A. Lieberman, III, M.D., M.P.H., a psychologist and a family physician teaching at the University of Medicine and Dentistry at the Robert Wood Johnson Medical School in New Jersey. They had filmed dozens of consultations of physicians who were very appreciated by their patients, as well as others with doctors who were much less valued. From these films, they distilled the essence of what helped make a strong human connection into an easy-to-learn technique.[1]

As many others did, I taught that method for years. My greatest surprise was to discover that it applied just as well to everyone—to my family, my friends, and even my colleagues—when they were going through a bad spell. These people were not consulting me as a psychiatrist. I was not necessarily available—nor did I always have the desire—to spend an hour going over the minute details of their story. With them, as well, I had to find the most effective and humane way to "make contact" and to help them feel better . . . in 10 minutes.

Dr. Stuart and Dr. Lieberman's method can greatly improve our capacity to relate to others—and thus, to feel better about ourselves—without needing to become a psychiatrist. We can use this technique to get closer to people who matter the most—our spouse, parents, children—as we have never learned to do in the past. By doing so, we strengthen our relationships. Because relationships have the power to regulate our emotional brains, this translates directly into protection from anxiety and depression—in fact, into well-being.

BATHEing the Heart

The technique consists of five steps you follow in fairly rapid succession. A useful mnemonic for remembering them is to think of BATHEing the other's heart.*

B for BACKGROUND. To connect with someone who is suffering, you must obviously find out first what happened to give them pain. This is what they will describe in answering your question, *"What happened to you?"*

What Dr. Stuart and Dr. Lieberman discovered is that one need not go into details; in fact, just the opposite. What is important is to get to the gist of what happened by listening with as little interruption as possible for 2 minutes, but not much longer. If 2 minutes do not seem like much, you will probably be surprised to learn that, on average, a doctor interrupts her patient after only 18 seconds.[2]

Still, allowing "only" 2 minutes also has a purpose. If you let the person talking to you run on for much longer, he is likely to get lost in details and you may never get to the heart of the matter. The essentials, after all, are never in the facts—they're in the feelings. Thus you must move on quickly to the second step, which is much more important.

---

*BATHE is taken from: Stuart, M. R., and Lieberman, J. A. III, *The Fifteen Minute Hour: Practical Therapeutic Interventions in Primary Care, 3rd Edition*. Philadelphia: Saunders, 2002.

A for AFFECT. The question you should now quickly raise is: *"And how does that make you feel?"* This may seem stilted to you, or embarrassingly obvious, but you'll be amazed what you'll learn. I taught this method to general practitioners in Kosovo after the horrors of the 1999 war. One day, one of my "trainees" was seeing a woman who complained of constant pain in her head, back, and hands, as well as sleeplessness and weight loss. The poor man ran down his mental list of all the possible diagnoses to be found in the medical encyclopedia, from syphilis to multiple sclerosis. I whispered in his ear to simply ask her, "What happened to you?"

Within a few seconds, she explained that she had not heard from her husband, who had been kidnapped by Serb militia several months earlier. She thought he must be dead. She probably had no one else to tell about it, since stories like that were so commonplace. We could certainly imagine what she must have felt. The trainee doctor hesitated to take the next step. It seemed too obvious. Asking the question about feelings somehow seemed almost insulting. Nevertheless, I encouraged him. He managed to get it out haltingly: "And how do you feel about this now?"

At that moment the woman finally dissolved in tears: "I am terrified, Doctor, terrified." He took her arm and let her cry a little. She had needed to do that for such a long time. Then he went on to the most important step of all.

T for TROUBLE. The best way to avoid drowning in emotion is to dive down deep, to the bottom, the hardest place, to the core of suffering. That is the only place where we can give the kick that will bring us back up to the surface.

Once again, the question seems discourteous, or "indecent," considering what the suffering of such an experience implies. Yet, it is the most effective of all the questions: *"And what troubles you the most now?"*

"Not knowing what to say to the children," the woman answered without a moment's hesitation. "I'd known for a long time it was going to happen. My husband and I had often talked about it. But the children . . . what can I do for the children?" She was racked by even more violent sobs. Her answer was not at all what I had anticipated when she spoke of her terror after losing her husband. But clearly all her emotions were centered on her children. If we had not asked her, we would never have guessed.

This question is magic because it helps focus the mind of the person in pain. She can start to pull her thoughts together around what hurts the most. Otherwise, abandoned to itself, her mind—our mind—would tend to fragment and feel overwhelmed.

I have experienced the powerful effect of this interaction myself. I was going through a difficult time after the end of a very important relationship in my life. I spent every evening alone and I felt sadness throughout my body. But I did not cry, I never cried. As many men have learned to do, I gritted my teeth and carried on. Life had not stopped because my heart was broken; there was always much to do.

One evening, a friend telephoned to find out how I was doing. I didn't like to dwell on the circumstances, because clearly, there was no satisfactory outcome. But my friend was a professor of pediatrics and she was also familiar with the importance of BATHEing the heart of someone in pain. When she asked me what troubled me the most, I suddenly saw the image of my son before my eyes—my son, who had come to help me move into my new apartment. I saw him at home, sad and vulnerable, probably gritting his teeth as well. And I was not there to help him.

At that moment I, too, literally dissolved in tears. All that unexpressed sadness had suddenly been channeled where it should have been from the beginning, into the tears and sobs that overcame me. The dam had burst. After a few minutes, I felt much better. Nothing was resolved, but I now knew what was causing a lot of my pain. And in this domain—my son's development—the future lay before me.

H for HANDLING. After giving voice to the emotions, you must capitalize on the energy that's concentrated on the principal source of the problem at that moment by asking, *"And what helps you the most to handle this?"* That question turns listeners' attention toward the resources around them that can help them to cope, to take charge.

Even when we see the people we love in their weakest moments, we must not underestimate their capacity to deal with the most difficult situations. What people often need most is help to get back on their feet, to collect their own resources. They often do not need us to solve their problems for them.

We all have trouble understanding and admitting that the men and women around us are stronger, more resistant, than we generally believe. That we *ourselves* are stronger and more resistant than we think. What I had to teach my doctor trainees—with some difficulty—is that we all need to learn in our emotional relationships as well. Instead of saying to ourselves, "Don't just stand there! Do something!" when someone expresses his feelings and his pain, we would do better to think, "Don't just do something! Stand there!" Because that is often the most useful role we can play. Our role consists of simply being there, being present, instead of offering a panoply of solutions and clumsily taking on the other person's problems.

The Albanian woman in Kosovo began by thinking for a moment. "My sister and my neighbors are all in somewhat the same situation," she said, "and we are together all the time. They are terrific with the children." That shared circumstance did not solve anything, obviously. But she saw a little more clearly where she could turn for her most pressing needs in the immediate future. And the mere fact of realizing more directly that this resource was there for her meant that she felt less lost. In my own case, what helped me was realizing that I could begin a new relationship with my son by taking matters into my own hands. Also, I knew I had a friend whom I could always talk to about everything, even if he lived far away. So I began calling him several times a week—in the evening, in fact, when loneliness weighed me down the most.

E for EMPATHY. Doctors who learn this method are able to connect with and help their patients very quickly. Part of that help is sending them off with the confidence that someone truly cares about them and the sense that they have an ally in their struggle. Of course, that's also your aim when you help a friend or loved one.

To finish this usually brief exchange, it's always useful to sincerely express the feelings you experienced as you listened to the other person. Pain is like a weight we carry around our neck. By talking about how you felt as you were listening to them, you are letting them know that you have shared their burden for a few minutes. At the end of the conversation, they will set out alone again with their heavy load. But because of those few minutes of carrying it together, they will feel a little less lonely on their path, and a little less daunted.

Usually, a few very simple words are enough. For example, *"That must be hard for you."* Or, *"I felt sad, too, as I listened to you. I'm so sorry that this happened to you."*[3]

Children who run to their mother when they hurt themselves know how important these words are, often much better than adults know. Obviously, their mother cannot do very much to make the pain go away. She's not a doctor or a nurse. But it is not just the pain that needs to be relieved; it's the loneliness, more than anything. Adults also need to feel less alone when they suffer.*

Our patient in Kosovo was not cured after 15 minutes in the doctor's office. But she was stronger and a lot less alone. As for her doctor, he felt more effective than if he had prescribed a battery of useless tests and medicines. He, too, like all the Kosovars I met there—Albanian or Serb—had suffered greatly and his emotions were almost as raw as

---

*I wish to thank Rachel Naomi Remen, M.D., for pointing out this distinction between pain and loneliness in her beautiful book, *Kitchen Table Wisdom* (Riverside Books, 1997).

those of the woman who was then leaving his office. But as I looked at him, I had the feeling that he felt better, too. He seemed more relaxed, more sure of himself. It was as if that brief exchange had helped them both grow; as if it had given them both a little dignity back. By relating to her, by showing her a bit of his humanity, he had also cared for himself. That is how our emotional brain develops, in successful exchanges like this one, even if they do not "heal" us instantly. Our emotional brain gains confidence in our ability to relate to others and be "regulated" by them, as it needs to be. And this confidence protects us from anxiety and depression.

Angela Talks to Her Mother

Psychiatrists and psychoanalysts often overlook the techniques of communication we have been discussing. They think of it as "common sense," not worthy of being researched or taught.

True, they should be common sense. But, as studies of practicing physicians show, and contrary to Descartes's opinion of the matter, common sense is often not very common; too often, it's certainly not a widely shared attribute. If parents always talked to their children in that way, if couples knew how to exchange constructive criticism and listen to each other with their hearts, if bosses knew how to respect their fellow workers, if common sense were indeed more common, we would not need to teach it. I found that when doing psychotherapy, it is often important to complement the treatment with very detailed instructions to patients. We all need guidance on how we can better regulate our emotional relationships with those who matter most to us. I have trouble understanding why we do not teach this more systematically.

Far from Kosovo, in a comfortable American city, one of my patients had to learn the fundamentals of effective emotional communication very fast to deal with the relationship that is often the most difficult of all—her relationship with her mother.

Angela was 55. At first glance, she appeared to have everything: a husband of 30 years who adored her; two handsome sons who were brilliant and, at the same time, particularly affectionate; a beautiful home in the nicest area of town. She had come to the United States from Italy at the age of 14. She had even done very well financially by creating and then selling a temporary employment agency.

Angela played tennis once or twice a week in a country club and she still enjoyed sensing a man's glance at her shapely figure. But beneath that smooth surface, Angela's inner self was in chaos. She was subject to anxiety attacks and woke up several times at night in a near panic. During the day, she sometimes hid away and cried. She constantly felt on the verge of suffocating.

Her doctor finally prescribed an anti-anxiety drug and an antidepressant. Angela had never taken medicine in her life. The idea of going on psychiatric medication struck her as inconceivable. She wanted to try something different.

When she came to see me, I was confident that with her intelligence and willpower we would soon bring her symptoms under control. Biofeedback sessions helped her master cardiac coherence. Several sessions of EMDR enabled her to clean out a large share of the heavy emotional baggage she had been carrying since her difficult childhood across two continents. She took steps to improve her eating habits. And, indeed, in a few weeks, she had made substantial progress. Yet Angela continued to have anxiety attacks from time to time, especially at night. She hadn't entirely rid herself of the sensation of suffocating that still occasionally beset her when she woke up in the morning.

When we reviewed her situation once again, I realized that she had greatly understated the violence of her emotional relationship with her mother, Marcella. After the death of her third husband, the old woman had left Naples to come and live with Angela in the United States.

Much as we may wish for an easy way to manage them, we cannot act as if extremely painful emotional relationships do not exist. We cannot stave them off with Prozac or even with the most effective natural treatments. Angela had no choice. She had to confront the situation.

Since coming to America, Marcella had refused to learn English or get a driver's license. Obviously, she was just plain bored. Interfering in her daughter's life seemed to be her principal pastime. With remarkable intelligence, she knew exactly how to make Angela feel guilty while all the while maintaining that she was not asking anything for herself. And whatever Angela did—that is, just about whatever Marcella asked—was never enough or never what she needed.

As it was out of the question to send her home alone to Italy or to put her in a retirement home where she would not have been able to talk to anyone, Marcella enjoyed an extraordinary position of power in the household. She needed to be taken care of. If she wasn't, she made everybody unhappy simply by sulking. Angela was now able to master her heart rate when her mother aimed one of her usual jabs at her. And thanks to EMDR, today's disputes no longer reawakened the pain and humiliation of physical punishment endured in her childhood. Still, she continued to undergo constant verbal and emotional abuse in her own home. Her Mediterranean culture, which emphasized submissiveness to parents, clearly had not prepared her to deal with such a difficult old mother.

Angela really only began to feel better when she agreed to systematically take charge of the emotionally volatile relationship with her mother. We drew up a list of the concessions she was willing to make and the limits she wanted to set. She was prepared to take her mother out to lunch and go shopping with her three times a week.

(That seemed a lot to me, but it was up to her to define what she found acceptable.)

On the other hand, Angela wanted peace in her household for an hour in the morning, after her husband had left for work. She also wanted an hour in the evening after he came back home. She did not think her mother would manage to stop railing at her. Marcella had always talked that way and, at 85, it was too late for that to change. On the other hand, Angela would no longer tolerate the threats of physical violence that her mother—as incredible as that may seem—continued to fling at her.

With her "STABEN" cue card in hand, we rehearsed the scene in which she would explain her needs to her mother. With my help, she had chosen the place and the timing for that conversation and the best way to broach the subject: "Dear Mother, you know how much it matters to me for you to be happy in my home and how important my role as your daughter is to me. There are certain things we need to talk over to make sure we can have the most harmony in the household." She had groped for the next words. Finally, she found a way to describe the behavior that bothered her, as well as her own emotions and needs: "Three things disturb me in your attitude. They prevent me from being as comfortable with you as I would like. First, when you interrupt me in my activities in the morning just after Luca leaves, I don't feel capable of doing everything at once. It's the time when I organize my day. I need to be alone for an hour. Then, when you join us as soon as Luca comes back from the office. It frustrates me to not have a moment with him before the family comes together again in the evening. I need an hour alone with him when he comes home. Finally, when you say things to me like 'I'm going to teach you a lesson.' Even if I know it isn't true, it frightens me and it's very unpleasant. I need to feel safe in my home and I need to know that there will never be any violence here."

The first day was hard. Angela had never confronted her mother like that! Because reality can be more sticky than role-playing, the discussion was not as straightforward as we had planned. However, Angela succeeded in letting Marcella know what she would like to do with her—the planned outings—and what she needed for herself. She asked her to cooperate with her. She also said that from that moment on, if she ever felt threatened, she would refuse to go out with Marcella for two days.

The first two weeks after that conversation were the most difficult. Naturally, Marcella tested the limits at the slightest opportunity. She found numerous compelling reasons to go to town in addition to the three weekly occasions she had agreed to. She had also, naturally, tested her daughter's resolve by threatening her on the third day. Angela called me practically every other day, but she held out. Even though her symptoms had somewhat worsened, she understood very well why and that worried her less.

After a month, the household atmosphere had calmed down considerably. Angela's symptoms had also subsided. That was when she finally felt capable of a greater emotional availability toward her mother who, after all, had had a difficult life, too. She simply used the BATHE method, to make sure she was listening systematically to the feelings hidden beneath Marcella's words and that she was helping her to express what bothered her most. Her mother was surprised by this attitude, but she soon enjoyed feeling listened to in that way. As she grew more comfortable with Angela's listening, she opened up about her own long, tumultuous life. Marcella told stories about her childhood in a poor village of Sicily. She talked about her first marriage—at 15—to a violent and alcoholic man. She described how she escaped to Naples by hiding in the hold of a boat. It was the stuff of novels. Angela kept supporting her through the stories, asking the same questions, again and again:

"And how did you feel when that happened?"

"And what was the most difficult thing for you about that?"

"And what helped you handle it?"

She also said, "That must have been hard for you, Mother," and her mother went on talking. Angela felt that, for the first time, her mother was taking her through the most important aspects of these old episodes. Her mother had never talked about her past with such detail and emotion. In some ways, they felt more connected to each other than they had in a long time—perhaps than they ever had.

Still, Marcella's character, for all that connectedness, had not really changed, and it probably never would. She remained an old, cantankerous person who required much emotional management. The difference was that Angela now had the sense of controlling her own life again. She had a new respect for herself and she could see very well that her mother also looked at her differently.

Black Belt and Beyond

Mastery of emotional communication is not achieved in a day or in a month. Not even in a year. A beginner in martial arts starts with a white belt and ends up with a black belt. Then come the endless refinements leading to higher titles called "dans" or "masters." But there is no "final master." You can always improve.

To me, the art of emotional communication is a little like that. It requires a mastery of inner energy that probably takes a whole lifetime to refine perfectly. After years spent looking into the matter—without any systematic training, it is true—I have the sense of being only a "brown belt" myself. Nevertheless, I have had enough experience to become convinced that it is tragic to go through life without applying yourself to the fundamental task of continually improving your own emotional communication. Even if that training can go on indefinitely, it's only one more reason to set to work immediately.

I like the story I heard once about Colbert, Louis XIV's great minister. France was severely lacking in sufficient boats to confront the growing power of England. There were not enough beech trees to make masts. Colbert called in the king's foresters and asked them to plant a forest. "But, Your Lordship," they answered, "it takes 100 years to grow beech trees tall enough for masts."

"Ah," said Colbert, "In that case . . . we must begin right away!"

Fortunately, the benefits of emotional communication can be felt a lot faster. Young doctors who learned about this method observed an almost immediate difference in their relationships with their patients and also in the energy they saved over the course of their long and difficult days. Developing that mastery is easier still when it's combined with a pursuit of heart rate coherence. Heart rate coherence stabilizes the emotional brain, and this appears to make us more receptive to our feelings as well as to the feelings of others. It helps us find words more easily and remain centered in our most authentic intentions.

I have discussed at great length the importance of regulating our emotions, and of the influence we exert on each other's feelings. After mastering our physiology, using methods focused on the body that are described in the first part of this book, managing communication is the next fundamental stage in healing the emotional brain. Still, there is another step in healing that has been largely neglected over the past 50 years in the West: what we do, not for ourselves, but for others. Each of us has a role in the community in which we live, beyond our own selves and even beyond our close relations. Humans are profoundly social animals. We cannot be happy, we cannot release the instinct to heal the core of our being, without finding meaning in our connection to the world around us—that is, in what we bring to others.

1 4

The Larger Connection

If I am not for myself, who will be for me?
And if I am for myself alone, then what am I?
And if not now, then when?

—HILLEL, *ETHICS OF OUR FATHERS*

Life is a struggle. And, it is a struggle that is not worth fighting, not merely for our own sake.

We are always looking for meaning beyond the weariness of being ourselves. We need a reason beyond mere survival to go on living. In *Wind, Sand and Stars*, Saint-Exupéry tells the pilot Henri Guillaumet's story. His plane had gone down in the Andes. For three days, he had walked straight ahead in the bitter cold. Then, he fell face down in the snow. The respite was unexpected, yet very welcome. But Henri realized that if he did not get up immediately, he would never get up again.

Exhausted to the depths of his being, he no longer wished to go on. He was drawn to a gentle, painless, peaceful death. In his thoughts, he bid goodbye to his wife and children. In his heart, he felt his love for them one last time. Then a new thought came to mind: If nobody found his body, his wife would have to wait 4 years to collect his life insurance.

Opening his eyes, he noticed a rock emerging from the snow 100 yards up ahead. If he dragged himself that far and onto the rock, his body would be a little more visible. Perhaps someone would spot it more quickly. Out of love for his family, he got up and started walking again. But now, he was carried forward by that love. He did not stop again. He went on, covering over 60 miles in the snow before reaching a village. Later he would say, " What I did, no beast on earth would have done." When his own survival was no longer sufficient motivation, his awareness of others—his love—gave him the strength to keep going.

Today we are in the midst of a worldwide trend centered on the self, on "personal development," on "self-psychology." Its key values are autonomy, independence, individual freedom, and self-expression. These values have become so central that even advertising executives use them to get us to buy the very same items that our neighbors already own, while convincing us that this will make us unique. "Be yourself," clothing and perfume advertisements cry out. "Express yourself," urges the advertisement for a brand of coffee. "Think different," a computer maker proclaims. Even the Army—hardly a model for independent thinking—adopted the message in order to attract young recruits. "Be all you can be," said its recruiting poster.

These values have been irrepressibly on the rise since the American and French Revolutions at the end of the 18th century. Naturally, they have done a great deal of good. These principles are at the core of the very idea of "liberty" that matters so much to us. But the further we move in that direction, the more clearly we see that this individual freedom has a cost.

The cost of this relentless pursuit of autonomy is isolation, suffering, and a loss of meaning. Never have we had as much freedom to part from spouses or partners who no longer suit us perfectly. The divorce rate is now approaching 50 percent in our societies. It is higher still in urban areas, where there are more opportunities to meet new partners.[1] Never before have we moved so often. (In the United States, according to some estimates, families move on average every 5 years.)

Released from family bonds, duties, obligations toward others, we have never been as free to seek our own way. But because of this same process, we can get lost and wind up alone. This growing alienation is probably one of the reasons why depression seems to have risen regularly in the West in the past 50 years.[2]

One of my friends was 37. He was a doctor who had emigrated from his country of birth and had lived alone until recently. For a long time, he had sought the meaning that was missing from his life. He turned to psychoanalysis, to a multitude of workshops on self-psychology, and then to antidepressants. He tried practically all of the different varieties. Then, one day, he told me, "In the end, the only time I stop asking myself existential questions is when my 2-year-old son puts his hand in mine and we go for a walk, even if it's only to pick up the paper!"

As it was for my friend, the most obvious source of meaning in our life is probably the love we feel for our partner and our children. But others' influence on and contribution to our own emotional balance does not stop with the nuclear family. In fact, the better integrated we are in a community we care about, and the stronger our feeling of playing a role in it that matters to others, the easier it is for us to overcome our feelings of anxiety, despair, and pointlessness.

I remember an old lady I used to see in her home because she was afraid to go out. She had emphysema and had to stay hooked up to her oxygen bottle all the time, but her principal problem was her depression. At 75, nothing interested her anymore. She felt empty and anxious, and she was now only waiting to die. Naturally, she slept

badly, had a poor appetite, and spent a good deal of her time complaining. I was struck, all the same, by her intelligence and her obvious competence. She had been an administrative assistant to an
important executive. There was an air of preciseness and natural authority about her that prevailed, despite her depression. One day I
told her, "I know you don't feel well at all and you need help. But you
are also someone whose skills could be extremely useful to other
people in need. What are you doing in your life to help others?" She
was very surprised that a psychiatrist—who was supposed to be
helping *her*—should ask such a question. Still, I could see her eyes
light up. She found the idea immediately engaging. She decided to
devote a little time to helping underprivileged children learn how to
read. It was not easy, all the more so because getting out and about
was truly complicated for her. Besides, not all of her pupils were
grateful—far from it—and some were downright hard to manage. But
this work took on a major role in her life. It gave her a goal, the
feeling she was useful. It anchored her, once again, in the community
from which she had been cut off by age and infirmity.

Camus understood this aspect of the soul, even if he did not talk
about it much in his philosophical essays. In *The Myth of Sisyphus*, his
description of the human condition is haunting. According to Camus,
our life basically consists of pushing a rock from the bottom to the
top of a mountain, where it will fall back down, and we will then
begin all over again. It would be an illusion to seek any meaning in
existence other than the fact that the rock is our rock, that it is
unique, and that we are responsible for it.

All the same, Camus says, as Sisyphus walks back down the mountain, we should think of him as happy. But this philosophy of the
"absurd" did not stop Camus from joining the Resistance during
World War II. He fought and was happy in the Resistance. Like many
men and women, he discovered a buoyancy in risking his life for a
cause much larger than himself—the fundamental joy of offering his

life for the lives of others. This meaning we find in our connection to others is not a cultural dictate or a rule of conduct imposed by society. It is a need emanating from the brain itself.

In the last 30 years, sociobiology has demonstrated that our very genes are altruistic. Our concern for others and the inner peace it brings are part of our genetic makeup.[3] Thus, there is nothing surprising in the fact that altruism is at the center of all great spiritual traditions.[4] Indeed, in his discussion of the neural origins of ethics, Dr. Damasio emphasized that altruism is, first of all, an *experience* in the body.[5] Joy in helping others is an emotion felt not only by Taoist and Hindu sages, and by Hebrew, Christian, and Moslem prophets, but also by millions of anonymous humans, many of them atheists.

Studies of people who are happier about their lives than others systematically point to two factors. Such people have close, stable emotional relationships with others, and they are involved in their community.[6] We have already talked at great length about emotional relationships, but what about larger social ties?

Involvement in the community means giving of ourself and of our time for a cause that offers no material benefit in return. This pursuit is one of the most effective activities when we are seeking to mitigate the feeling of emptiness that often goes with depressive states. And, luckily for us, we don't have to risk our life or join the Resistance to reap these benefits.

Bringing a bit of light into the lives of elderly people who are shut in; working in an animal shelter; volunteering to help at the neighborhood school; participating in the town council or the company union—all of these activities draw us out of our own little isolating sphere and make us feel connected to the spheres of others. And, in the end, we feel less anxious and less depressed. The founder of modern sociology, Emile Durkheim, was the first to demonstrate this. One hundred years ago, in his groundbreaking book, *Suicide*, he showed that people who are the least "integrated" members of their community are those who commit suicide most often.[7] More recently, modern sociologists have found not only that people who participate in community activities are happier, but that they are also in better health and live longer than others. A study published in the *American Journal of Cardiology* confirms this. The research concerns a group of elderly poor people. It found that with the same health conditions, the mortality rate of subjects who do volunteer work devoted to others is 60 percent lower than that of people who do not.[8]

The effects of volunteer work on health were also analyzed in *Science*, the best-known scientific journal. This study concludes that volunteer activities are one of the best guarantees of a longer life. Volunteering may be an even better safeguard than maintaining low blood pressure, keeping down cholesterol, or giving up cigarettes.[9] The pleasure of being connected to others, the feeling of involvement in a social group, is a remarkable remedy for the emotional brain and thus for the body as well.

The Austrian psychiatrist Victor Frankl survived Nazi concentration camps. In *Man's Search for Meaning*, his moving book based on his experience, he explains what enabled some prisoners to hold on, in spite of it all.[10] His observations do not have scientific value; however, his conclusions are similar to those of the research studies. Survival in a cold and indifferent world forces us to find a meaning in our existence, to connect to something. Much like President Kennedy's famous admonition, his advice in desperate circumstances is to ask not what life can do for us, but to always ask instead what we can do for life. This outlook may simply mean doing our job with more generosity, keeping in mind how it contributes to others' lives. Or it may mean giving a little of our time, once a week, to a cause, a group, or simply to another person, or even to an animal we are fond of.

Mother Teresa was probably the undisputed champion of charity in action in the 20th century. She said, "Don't look for spectacular actions. What is important is the gift of yourselves. It is the degree of love you insert in your deeds."[11] Nor is it necessary to be perfectly at ease with yourself to be able to give of yourself. The psychologist Abraham Maslow was the founder of a new school of psychology often referred to as "the Human Potential Movement." At the end of his study of healthy, psychologically balanced people, he concluded that the final stage of personal development comes when the "actualized" individual begins to turn toward others. He even talks about becoming a "servant," while insisting on the importance of self-fulfillment. "The best way to become a better helper is to become a better person. But one necessary aspect of becoming a better person is *via* helping other people. So one can and must do both simultaneously."[12]

A century after Durkheim, 30 years after Frankl and Maslow, modern studies in physiology have confirmed their insights and observations. When a computer measures cardiac coherence, we observe that the simplest and fastest way for the body to establish coherence is to experience feelings of gratitude and tenderness toward others.[13] When we sense in a visceral way—emotionally—our connection to those around us, our physiology automatically achieves coherence. At the same time, when we help our physiology bring about coherence, we open the door to new ways of taking in the world around us. This virtuous circle described by Maslow is the gateway to realizing the self—without stress, anxiety, or depression.

15

Getting Started

Standing on the Pont Neuf, in the heart of Paris, I watch the Seine flow between large white stones. On the bank, a man is fishing with his son. The little boy just caught a fish and his eyes are gleaming with joy. I remember a long walk with my father along that same river, when I was that little boy's age. He was telling me about my grandfather who used to swim in the Seine. But, he added, the river was now so polluted that no one could swim in it anymore. Even the fish had disappeared from the water.

Today, only 35 years later, the fish have come back. Perhaps one can even swim in the Seine again. All it took was to stop polluting the river, and the river took care of itself. Given the chance, and enough time, it purified its waters. Rivers and streams are alive. Like us, they tend toward "homeostasis," toward balance. They have, in fact, an instinct to heal.

Like all living things, rivers are in a constant exchange with their environment: air, rain, earth, trees, algae, fish, and man. And that exchange of life creates more order, more organization, and, in the end, more purity. Only still waters become brackish. They drift into chaos. Death is, indeed, the opposite of life: There is no longer any exchange with the outside. In death, the creation of balance and the constant rebuilding of order that defines life yields to decomposition.

But as long as natural forces are at work in life, they guard against decomposition. They strive toward order, coherence, and even purity. Aristotle thought that every life-form had an energy, a force, that he called "entelechy" or autocompletion.[1] He even talked of a "duty" of all living things to reach autocompletion. A seed or an egg contains within itself the force that will transform it into a vastly more complex organism, whether a flower, a tree, a chicken, or a human being. That process of autocompletion is not only physical—in human beings, it extends itself through the development of maturity and wisdom. Carl Jung and Abraham Maslow made the same observation. Jung was fascinated by the process of "individuation," which pushes human beings toward ever more maturity and serenity. Maslow called it "self-actualization." They referred to self-healing and autocompletion as the natural purpose of life itself.[2]

The treatment methods described in this book all share the aim of strengthening these mechanisms that apply to all life-forms—from single cells to entire ecosystems, human beings included. Each method, in its own way, supports the body's constant attempt to foster coherence, to recover its balance. Because of this, the different methods work in synergy: It's not necessary to choose one at the exclusion of any other. To the contrary, they all strengthen each other. For example, as I discovered while I was researching the scientific literature while writing this book, every single one of these methods happens to strengthen the balance of the parasympathetic nervous system. This branch of the autonomic nervous system appeases and soothes many different functions in the body and in the mind. It is therefore easier to experience the mood-enhancing and stress-relieving benefits of practicing heart rate coherence if one also exercises, eats more omega-3 fatty acids, or eliminates the traces of old traumatic emotional experiences through EMDR, because all of these help restore the balance between the sympathetic and the parasympathetic nervous system. By doing so, they help reset the emotional brain and keep it functioning in an optimal range.[3]

Modern medicine has lost the very concept of synergy. The single greatest transformation in the history of medicine took place in the 1940s. For the first time, terrifying and mortal diseases could be defeated with a specific and reliable treatment. Pneumonia, syphilis, gangrene, tuberculosis, all yielded to antibiotics. These new medicines were so effective that everything that had been essential to medicine until then suddenly seemed irrelevant: With antibiotics, as long as the patient took her pills, healing seemed to follow. It didn't matter whether doctors cared or not, it didn't matter much what the patient ate, it didn't even matter whether she wanted to get better. She took the antibiotic and the disease retreated.

These old pillars of medicine—the doctor-patient relationship, healthy nutrition, the patient's attitude, and so on—looked like outdated and misguided concepts. From this fantastic advance, a new medicine was born in the Western world, a medicine that no longer took into account the patient's history, his or her web of relationships, the strength of his or her life force, of his or her self-healing mechanisms. This new and purely mechanical perspective on patients and diseases promptly generalized to all of medicine, well beyond the realm of infectious diseases.

Today, most of the teaching delivered in Western medical schools focuses on diagnosing specific illnesses in order to choose a specific treatment. This approach works remarkably well for acute conditions: surgical removal of the appendix for an appendicitis, penicillin for a pneumonia, a corticosteroid for an asthma attack, and so on. However, the "specific treatment" approach falls short of any true healing for chronic illnesses. In chronic conditions, the modern Western approach generally helps only with crises, such as an asthma attack, or a heart attack; it does not help with the underlying condition.

Take the example of a heart attack. A patient comes in to an emergency room (ER) on the verge of death—pale, nauseous, suffocating, with crushing pain in her chest. The ER doctors know exactly what to do: Within minutes, oxygen flows through nasal prongs, nitroglycerin dilates her vessels, a beta-blocker slows down her heart rate, aspirin prevents additional clotting, and morphine relieves her pain. Less than 10 minutes later, the woman's life has been saved. She can breathe normally, she can talk to her family, she can even smile. In many ways, this is medicine at its best.

However, for all the drama of this powerful intervention, the underlying disease—the progressive clogging of the woman's arteries from inflamed plaques of cholesterol—has not been touched. To this day, the most effective interventions to treat the underlying illness are deceptively nontechnical. I almost want to say "nonmodern." They consist of a combination of stress management, exercise, and better nutrition. The synergy between these lifestyle changes can induce a profound cleansing of the arteries, much like the cleansing of a formerly polluted river.

Exactly the same is true for anxiety and depression. They are *chronic* illnesses, not at all like acute infections or broken arms. A chronic illness arises through complex interactions between body systems that have started to malfunction. It is also fed by some form of "pollution" form the outside, be it in the form of maladapted nutrition, traumatic events, or chronically painful relationships. After years of maladaptive functioning and poisoning from the outside, it would be naive to think that a single intervention or even a single type of intervention could systematically rebalance the system or set it on the path to self-healing. All practitioners who work with chronic illnesses, whichever type they are, agree on this point. A synergy between several interventions is the only way to reverse a long-standing condition that has set itself into the body. Even the most entrenched psychotherapists and biological psychiatrists are forced to admit that combining psychotherapy and medication is more effective than either alone for chronic forms of depression. This was recently confirmed by a large and impressive study from several university centers, published in the *New England Journal of Medicine*.[4]

To overcome a chronic illness, we need to capitalize on all the mechanisms of self-healing to which we have access. We need to build, through several interventions, a treatment synergy greater than the momentum of the illness itself. This is the spirit in which I presented the different methods discussed in this book. Even if each one of these methods has been studied individually and found to be effective, the most effective treatment is to find the combination that is best adapted to each person, the combination that has the greatest chance of transforming his pain and giving his life its energy back.

Building Your Own Plan

We have reviewed many tools that reach into the depths of the emotional brain and help restore its coherence. So, concretely, how should one get started? In our Center for Complementary Medicine at the University of Pittsburgh, we settled on simple rules to help choose the best combination for each patient. We moved each patient through a step-by-step process, with each successive treatment building on the next. The principles are the following:

1. Practice Heart Coherence

The first priority is to learn how to control our emotional being. Throughout our lives, we all develop our preferred method of self-soothing during times of increased stress. Most of the time, we are encouraged to practice one or the other because somebody is making money selling it, not because it is particularly effective or nourishing to our emotional balance. Perhaps we've learned to rely on chocolate, ice cream, beer, whiskey, or cigarettes whenever we feel the first pangs of "stress," or perhaps we simply retreat into the anesthetic effects of television. These are, by far, the most common options used when life isn't delivering what we want or expect.

If we've turned to conventional medicine for help, these everyday little helpers have most likely been upgraded to anti-anxiety medicines such as Valium, Ativan, or Xanax, or to antidepressants. In the 1960s, almost every medical journal in the United States featured an ad for Librium, the predecessor of Valium. It said, in big letters, "Librium: Whatever the problem is!" Today, we are more likely to be told to take Prozac, Zoloft, or Paxil than an anti-anxiety medication, but the spirit is, in many ways, the same. The message that accompanies these medications is still that they are presumed to work "whatever the problem is." This tenacious belief is one of the reasons they are among the most prescribed and most profitable medicines today.

In place of a physician, you—or your children—may receive advice from a group of slightly lost and confused friends, which may lead to much more drastic alternatives as the preferred self-soothing methods: Marijuana, cocaine, or heroin are the street versions of the mother's little helper.

Obviously, whenever possible, one would be in much better shape to capitalize on the self-healing abilities of the emotional brain and of the body to reach a balance between cognition, emotions, and a sense of confidence in what life can provide. In Pittsburgh, we encouraged our patients to discover their ability to control their own cardiac coherence and to then use that state whenever they are confronted with the inevitable challenges of existence instead of turning to cigarettes or chocolate. Learning to enter into coherence can replace other less healthy, and often less effective, self-soothing methods to manage stress on the spot. To learn to maximize your heart coherence:

- To begin with, reread the description of heart coherence training on page 52 and start practicing the breathing and mental focus technique at least 10 to 15 minutes every night before going to bed. This is a good time to practice because most people can use a bit of help in the transition from a hectic home or work environment to turning inside oneself for the night. This is a wonderful time to reconnect with our own inner core and let ourselves experience gratitude and warmth toward that body, that heart, that carried us through all the ups and downs of the day, as it does every day, as it has done since our very first day.

  Practicing in this way, before going to bed, at a time when there should be no other demands on you, can only deepen your sleep and therefore more than make up for the few minutes required to make the connection and enjoy the experience. In addition, it helps you remember what you *can* feel like inside when you make an effort to be connected with your heart. And it is the very practice of this feeling that makes it easier to bring it on when you need it the most—in situations of stress!

- The most important step is to practice entering into coherence whenever things in your life are going wrong and pushing your physiology into chaos. What will make the greatest immediate difference in how you feel is your ability to generate coherence inside your heart and your mind precisely when things are not going right: when you're stuck in traffic, when you're being yelled at by an angry driver, when your child comes home with a terrible report from school, or when a coworker is sneering at an idea you just presented. In all of these situations, we have only two choices: be stuck with it *and* feel terrible inside, or be stuck with it and experience coherence.

- Many people can experience the light feeling of relaxation, or warmth, or lightness, inside their chest that comes with coherence without a computer biofeedback system. However, some feel much more comfortable with the exercise if they can prove to themselves that they are indeed producing coherence in their heart rhythm. For that purpose, it is possible to buy software that runs on most personal computers to test yourself and also see if you're making progress in how easily you can bring on coherence from one week or one month to the next. (Addresses for purchasing such computer packages are at the end of the book in the Resources section on page 239.)

• Finally, some organizations offer training in heart rate coherence. (See the Resources section on page 239.)

2. ADDRESS PAINFUL MEMORIES

The next step, whenever possible, is to identify past events that continue to trigger painful emotions when you think about them in the present. If talking or just thinking about something that happened in the past brings up tears, or stirs up strong feelings of anger, then it hasn't been resolved. Any memory that you actively try *not* to think about is generally one that has left a painful scar in your emotional brain.

Many patients tend to underestimate the importance of past pains. They do not see how old wounds continue to condition how they experience life, constantly kindling the sting—or perhaps simply reducing their ability to experience pleasure. Yet, a few sessions of EMDR are often enough to clean out the consequences of old sufferings and to give rise to a new and more harmonious perspective on life.

• For this purpose, you should consider contacting a thoroughly trained licensed psychotherapist in your area. A list of qualified practitioners is provided through the Web site of the EMDR Institute, at www.EMDR.com. You should then ask your family doctor or your friends about whom they would recommend as a good therapist from that list. As with all other forms of psychotherapy, EMDR will work best in the hands of a caring and well-trained therapist in whom you feel comfortable confiding.

- You should also inquire whether your therapist is covered by your health plan. Most insurance companies will cover EMDR sessions. However, some special arrangements may have to be made if the therapist feels that, in your situation, 90-minute sessions would be most appropriate, as they often are.

3. Manage Conflict and 4. Enrich Relationships

After working on the past, it is important to identify chronic conflicts in the most important relationships of the present: both at home, with parents, children, partners, brothers, and sisters, and at work, with our boss, coworkers, or employees. These relationships condition our emotional ecosystem. If they continuously pollute the flow of our emotional life, they end up blocking our mechanisms of adaptation and self-healing.

On the other hand, if they are purified, we can be set on a path toward balance and internal harmony. Occasionally, resolving old traumatic wounds will be enough to allow our relationships to find a new life. Once freed from the ghosts of the past, it is often possible to find completely new—and healthier—ways of relating to those who matter in our life.

Learning to be an effective emotional communicator—through nonviolent assertive communication—is a direct and powerful way to bring more balance to our relationships. We should all be constantly striving toward more effective ways of communicating with others. Beyond practicing the techniques described in this book, there are helpful workshops for practicing better communication techniques. When the most important conflicts lie in the realm of close personal relationships, the problem requires the intervention of a couple or family therapist.

- In order to begin learning how to effectively assert yourself through healthy emotional communication, reread the section, "The Six-Point Cue Card for Handling Conflict," page 188. Copy the STABEN method onto a card and practice it regularly, beginning with people you trust and branching out into other relationships, once you've gained your confidence. Just as it did for the father in the story, eventually, using this method will become second nature.
- To enrich and further strengthen your relationships, reread the section, "BATHEing the Heart" on page 195, and copy down the BATHE acronym on a card as well. Start with a relationship in which you find it a challenge to slow down and listen; it's likely that this will be the one in which you'll see the greatest benefits very quickly. The first time, you may even want to practice on the phone—no one will notice you're using a card.
- For more help in contacting a therapist or attending a workshop in your area, see the Resources, page 239.

5. MAXIMIZE OMEGA-3S

Almost anyone can benefit from a change in diet that restores the necessary balance between omega-3 fatty acids and other sources of fat. We know today that the "Cretan Diet"—which is particularly rich in omega-3 fatty acids—can restore healthy cardiac function. New research is now showing that it can positively influence cardiac variability and battle stress and depression as well.

Everybody should at least consider rebalancing their diet by increasing its fish content (or vegetarian sources of omega-3 fatty acids) and by reducing unhealthy fats. Before taking a casually prescribed antidepressant, I think people should consider whether they would benefit from taking supplements of omega-3, above and beyond changes in diet.

- Begin by adding some of the foods high in omega-3s, listed on page 139.
- Consider adding a fish oil supplement to your regimen; for recommended brands, see the Resources section, page 239; start with 1 gram of EPA (eicosapentaenoic acid) (probably the most important of the omega-3s for depression) per day. There are very few side effects, aside from occasional loose stools or gastric upset, if you start with a dose that is too high for your stomach to handle. If you experience a fishy aftertaste, you should make sure to take the supplement at the beginning of a meal or at night when you're going to bed.
- Check with your doctor if you are taking Coumadin (or its generic equivalent, warfarin), aspirin therapy, or any other medications that affect blood clotting, as omega-3s can also reduce clotting. This may require a reduction in your medication.
- Existing data suggest that omega-3s are important for fetal development and help prevent postpartum depression. However, it is always important to be extra careful when taking anything during pregnancy (especially the first 3 months) or while breastfeeding. So, if you plan on becoming pregnant, or if you are breastfeeding, you should seek the advice of your doctor about taking an omega-3 supplement and about the type of supplement that you are considering.

6. GET "HIGH" ON EXERCISE

Recommending a regular program of physical exercise has become a common suggestion from all kinds of physicians. However, this is very rarely done for people who suffer from anxiety and depression, even though the benefits are clearly established. This option is open to everyone, and all it requires is an investment of 20 to 30 minutes three times a week.

- Remember, it's the regularity, not the intensity, that matters for stress and anxiety reduction.
- Pick an activity you consider "play" or at least very enjoyable. Don't force yourself to take on jogging if you prefer swimming. And don't put too much pressure on yourself to perform. The only "inadequate" exercise is no exercise at all! Even if you start with 10 minutes of slow trotting, this will be considerably better than doing nothing. Slow down to a walk as soon as you're out of breath. You can pick up the pace when you can breathe comfortably again. Over a few weeks of regularly practicing in this way, you will feel more and more comfortable and notice that you no longer need to stop where and when you used to. But it will take a few weeks. Be patient and kind to yourself.
- If possible, join a group of like-minded exercisers who can both motivate you and help you out of a funk. Of course, the mistake would be to join a group of people who are all much more fit than you are and who may make you feel discouraged. This is not about comparing yourself to anybody, but about finding support and motivation to continue several times a week, week after week.
- Overall, success with an exercise program is about the three P's: get Pleasure, with People, and Persist.

7. WAKE UP TO THE SUN

In the same vein as exercise, we should all consider making another noninvasive change to our habits, to allow our bodies to benefit from waking up more peacefully in the morning. All that is required to reset our biological clock every day is to replace our raucous alarm clock with the gentle waking of a dawn simulator.

- The first thing to do is to keep a regular schedule: go to bed at pretty much the same time every day and wake up around the same time. Studies of patients who have ups and downs in their mood show that a regular sleep schedule helps them remain even and keep their balance.[5] This can be hard when you feel stressed by how many things need to be attended to in your life, or when you feel depressed and your sleep is affected. Yet, it's an important step in bringing your biological rhythms back in sync.

- Then, try to benefit from the regulating influence of waking up with the light of dawn. During the summer, you can try to simply keep your curtains open (though that does not give you control over the time of day when dawn will start waking you. This will change a little bit every day).

- To get control over when dawn wakes you up, you need to get a dawn simulator. Such devices are widely available; see Resources, page 239, for some affordable options.

- In order for the dawn simulator to control your wake-up time (and not the natural daylight, in case that's earlier than your wake-up time), you will need to make sure that your curtains or blinds can block out the outdoor sunlight completely. Of course, that's not a problem in the wintertime, when we all tend to wake up earlier than the sun.

- You should schedule your light to turn on 30 or 45 minutes before your appointed wake-up time. You can experiment with the duration that works best for you (though not all dawn simulators give you the same range of choices).

- For all of their benefits, dawn simulators don't allow you to cut down on your required amount of sleep. You will still need to get enough sleep in order to feel refreshed the next day.

8. TAP INTO YOUR MERIDIANS

Admittedly, acupuncture represents a larger investment of time and finances than some of the other methods. We have been recommending acupuncture treatments mostly to patients who not only have depression or anxiety but who also suffer from physical pain or other physical problems that are known to respond to this modality. In such cases, the Chinese needles can address both problems at the same time. When physical pain is a constant burden on the body, overcoming depression is very difficult, but since acupuncture has shown results with both types of symptoms, it can be very helpful in these circumstances.

- See Resources, page 239, for information on how you can find a
  qualified practitioner near you. If you try to choose from a listing,
  remember to ask your physician or your friends about which one
  they would recommend.

  Good practitioners take time to do a full assessment of your
  history and your symptoms before they start stimulating your
  body with needles. They should be gentle and caring, and the
  insertion of needles should be practically pain free. Furthermore,
  they should be ready to work in cooperation with your conventional physician and medications. Beware of acupuncturists who
  promise too much or of those who try to steer you away from
  conventional approaches that have worked for you.

9. SEEK A LARGER CONNECTION

Finally, for most of us, a true sense of peace can be reached only once we have found how we can contribute to the community that we live in and feel comfortable with the role we have in it. Even beyond this, many find solace in the sensation—a physical experience in the body—of being connected, not only to others around us, but to an even greater mystery that transcends us. Those who have the good fortune of being connected in this way often feel propelled much be- yond a simple well-being: They feel that they draw their energy from what gives meaning to life itself, in good times and in hardships.

- Take some time to think about the places and people among
  whom you feel most "at home" outside of your immediate family,

those whose very existence makes the world seem to be a better place to you. This place or group may be a park in your city, or a national forest, a local school, a soup kitchen, a choir, a church or temple, perhaps an animal shelter, or even a salsa dancing group.

- Are there any specific goals, beliefs, or philosophies in which you truly believe? Something that you think can make life on our planet better? It could be about literacy, but also about wildlife conservancy, or about feeling closer to the mystery of the universe and the connection of all things.

- If you can combine this essential feeling of "at homeness" with ideas that you really believe in, and find an activity or a group that embody both of these, then think of how you can get involved, or how you can contribute by being the person you are, in your own town, within your own means.

- Check the Resources section, page 239, for more ideas about how you can connect with your larger community, however you choose to define it.

Epilogue

As every French boy does at 16, I read *The Stranger* by Albert Camus while I was finishing high school. I remember very clearly the sense of being totally puzzled by the book.

Camus was right: This is all absurd. We all float haphazardly through existence, bump into random people who are equally disoriented, do things that we don't understand but that turn out to determine the course of our lives, and eventually die without having figured out what happened. If we are lucky, we may maintain a sense of integrity and pride from the fact that we are at least aware of the absurdity of the whole thing (and, if we are French, a certain disdain for those who do not display such awareness!). There is nothing else to expect.

At 41, after years spent tending to the pain and confusion of women and men from all over the world, I look at *The Stranger* quite differently. It seems clear to me now that the hero Camus chose to describe lived in disconnection from his emotional brain. He had no sense of inner life, to which he had never turned: He was unable to connect with pain or sorrow at his mother's funeral, nor joy and attachment in the presence of his girlfriend. He certainly derived no meaning for his existence from his dedication to a community (this is perfectly captured by the title of the book itself—the hero is, above all, a "stranger"). He also actively denied himself any opportunity to experience a connection with the transcendent.

Yet, after millions of years of evolution, our emotional brain is wired to crave four aspects of life, precisely the four that the stranger denied himself: a sense of connection to our body and inner states; intimacy with a few select human beings; a solid role in our community; and a sense of connection with the mystery of life. Estranged from these, we search in vain for a purpose outside of ourselves, in a world in which we have become . . . a stranger.

As neurologist Dr. Damasio brilliantly explained, 50 years after Camus, what gives depth and a sense of direction to our lives are the waves of feeling that arise from these sources of meaning to animate our body and our emotional neurons. And so, it is by cultivating each one of these crucial, elemental aspects of our own humanity that we can finally release the force that we were all born with: our instinct to heal.

Acknowledgments

When I am asked how long it took me to write this book, I answer truthfully: a few months and, before that, all my life. A book is the product of all those who contributed to developing the author's ideas—including schoolteachers who still frequently come to mind—as much as of those who contributed to his emotional development. Among them all, I can thank only a very small number here.

First, I must begin by expressing my gratitude to Beverly Spiro and Lewis Mehl-Madrona, two exceptional practitioners of the new medicine, alongside whom I had the chance to study and work. Their humanity, their effectiveness, and their constant encouragements forced me to open my thinking to many new ways of practicing my profession. Together, we founded the Center for Complementary Medicine at Shadyside Hospital. Patricia Bartone, a faithful friend and colleague at the Center, also helped me to make the break when the time came for me to return to my native country. Friends who are capable of helping you leave them are rare. And then there are all the members of the team—Denise Mianzo, Denise DiTommaso, Gayle Dentino, J. A. Brennan—as well as the practitioners who taught me so much and who continued to encourage and help me long after I left the Center. I owe all of them my appreciation. Jo Devlin, who taught the residents in Family Medicine together with me, gave me many of my ideas about how to improve doctor-patient relationships and about practicing psychotherapy with people in dire circumstances.

The hospital librarian, Michele Klein-Fedyshin, is a remarkably creative and efficient woman. Thanks to her almost daily e-mails, which reached me when I was working on my manuscript in the heart of the countryside—surrounded only by fields and cows—I was able to assemble the documents that provide the foundation for the ideas set forth in this book. Through her, I also wish to thank my former colleagues at Shadyside Hospital for their unfailing support, and especially Randy Kolb, my family doctor; Fred Rubin, chairman of the department of internal medicine; and David Blandino, chairman of the department of family and community medicine. Each of them has been a model for me, as a human being and as a doctor.

I would like to hail the open-mindedness of the dean of the School of Medicine of the University of Pittsburgh, Arthur Levine. Perhaps it was the admiration we shared for 19th-century Russian literature that was a determining factor in the tolerance he exercised toward a center for complementary medicine, in a university known to be a prestigious and successful center of orthodoxy. In France, Jean Cottraux, director of the department for the treatment of anxiety disorders at the Neurological Hospital in Lyon, is an unfailing source of wisdom about psychiatry. I wish to express my deep appreciation to him for his hospitality, his support, and his advice, even though he may not always agree with the views I express here.

All of the ideas that came together in this book began with my encounter with Jonathan Cohen, who now directs the Center for the Study of Mind, Brain and Behavior at Princeton University. It was a most unlikely meeting. We had both come to Pittsburgh, of all places, straight from our training in psychiatry, to study computer models of the brain. I was instantly fascinated with Jonathan's wit, his warm and fragile smile, and the amazing sharpness of his mind. We practically did not leave each other for another 8 years after that, and we learned together about failure and success, separation, loneliness, and the warm glow of friendship in the tunnel of life, just as much as we learned about the brain.

I have to thank the current and former chairmen of the department of psychiatry at the University of Pittsburgh, David Kupfer and Thomas Detre. Twenty years ago, they believed in me enough to invite a foreign student to come to Pittsburgh to pursue these interests. They unfailingly supported my pursuits from that day on, wherever these interests took me, even when they departed completely from theirs.

Herbert Simon, my thesis director, and Jay McClelland, who advised me all along, were role models of formidable stature who taught me everything I know about audacity and rigor in scientific thinking.

On the clinical side of my life, no other thinker has impressed me as much as Francine Shapiro, the creator of EMDR (Eye Movement Desensitization and Reprocessing). Francine exudes intelligence, sensitivity, courage, and determination in the face of considerable adversity and, at times, calumny. I also want to salute her respect for science and empirical examination of her method, which is what convinced me that it was worth exploring.

My analyst, Judith Schachter, allowed me to trust myself enough to pursue my own ideas. She was generous, and warm, and I will never forget the day when she transgressed the orthodoxy—even though she had become president of the American Psychoanalytic Association—and accepted my request to hold my hand when I asked her if she would, because I was sad and I needed her to.

Olga Tereshko, with her Russian soul, her strength, her passion, her humor, and her incisive intelligence, has given me tremendous love and has profoundly influenced my ideas on human nature. She also gave me the courage and support necessary to leave the trodden path of conventional academic success at a time when I was full of hesitations.

Among my family members, my son Sacha's small hand held in mine has given me the best reason in the world for writing. My brother Edouard has been a steadfast companion whose insights into these pages have been among the most penetrating and useful. My brother Franklin's advice on communication and relations to the media has kept me from making all of the expected mistakes of a beginner. And the strength, determination, and wit of my brother Emile have been a model for a long time. My mother, Sabine, has kept watch and helped steady the course of my life, a role at which she excels. My Uncle Jean-Louis organized my return to France with loving kindness and, on occasion, highly effective exhortations. He taught me to write for the lay public and I also owe him my thanks for suggesting the original title for this book (*Guérir*, which means, "to cure"). I am grateful to my Aunt Bernadette and her son Diego for their ingenuity and family loyalty in an alarming situation that could have prevented me from finishing the manuscript on time. The ever-faithful Liliane, who understands everything, thinks of everything, and has been organizing the details of family life for the last 40 years, enabled me to concentrate on my project. Annick, who helped raise me with her gentle ways, has also contributed to family life for just as long. Finally, Anatole and Tamara Tereshko, my son's grandparents, gave immensely of their time and energy to take care of Sacha while I was busy discovering new aspects of my profession.

The "midwife" who assisted the birth—the actual writing—of this book was Madeleine Chapsal, in her calm, hospitable country houses,

"La Sauterie," in the heart of France, and "La Maison Blanche," on the little paradise of the Isle of Ré. Madeleine has been encouraging me to write since I was 15. I still remember her comments on my high school graduation exam, an essay on the existential philosopher Merleau-Ponty. It was in Merleau-Ponty's room at "La Sauterie" that I wrote the first lines of this book. And during those shared weeks of forced isolation, we ate lots of fish and laughed a lot.

My friends Benoît Mulsant, Maurice Balick, Heidi Feldman, Tamara Cohen, Nikos Pediaditakis, and Lotti Gaffney have served as sounding boards, each in their own way, for the ideas expressed here. Their patience and loyalty, despite my flighty and absent-minded displays of friendship, have been a precious gift. Heidi's strength, courage, generous vision of medicine, and sheer power of conviction may have saved our fledgling center during its difficult beginnings.

My Sunday evening card game companions—earlier in Pittsburgh, now in Paris—are one of the reasons why it is good to be alive. All my thanks to Christine Gonze, Madjid, Youssef, Isabelle, Benoît, Géraldine, and Nicolas. I rediscovered the "call" of my native country after 20 years of voluntary exile when we met for the first time in Pittsburgh, purely for the pleasure of the game and for laughs. It helped me see more clearly what was missing from my sometimes ascetic life and what was essential to healing the soul—my own, in any case.

At the key moments of its creation, Roy and Susie Dorrance, and through them the spirit of their daughter, Emilie, who died at the age of 24, believed in this book. I have never known people who, on such slight acquaintance, have been as generous as they have been to me. Their kindness is engraved in my heart. I only hope I am worthy of the confidence they have shown me. I am grateful to Sonny Richards, one of the last Lakota shamans. The spiritual son of the great Fool's Crow, he is an incarnation of traditional Native American medicine, based on the exploration of emotions, community integration, and sacred rituals.

My gratitude also goes to Michael Lerner—probably one of the most fascinating American intellectuals of our time. He is deeply committed to a life of action and is always ready to fight the crucial battles facing our society. Thank you, Michael, for looking me in the eyes and saying, "You must write this book."

I am greatly indebted to Carol Mann, my agent in New York. First, because I got to tell my friends and myself that I actually had "an agent in New York"(!) when this book didn't even exist, but more importantly, because her superb judgment and her professionalism allowed me to transform the vague ideas of a practicing physician into an actual, readable book. I would also like to mention the dedicated and steadfast enthusiasm of my editor at Rodale—the warm Mariska van Aalst—and the commitment and encouragement of Amy Rhodes, who was one of the first publishers to see an exciting project in what was only an incomplete proposal.

Without the patience and organizational skills of Delphine Pécoul, my assistant, and the unrelenting friendship of Daniele Stern, who put together all the missing pieces of this project in the last few weeks before the deadline, I would not have had the freedom to concentrate on the essentials.

Finally, I would like to salute the spirit of my father, Jean-Jacques, which infuses every page of this book. I remember, as a child, seeing him at his desk in the family house in Normandy, working throughout the summer when he wrote *The American Challenge*. With its new and provocative ideas, that book opened up minds the world over. I was sitting at the same desk when I drew the first outline of this *Instinct to Heal*. I have not had to revise it a single time since.

Island of Ré, August 2003

Resources

For the most recent information, please refer to the Web site www.instincttoheal.org, which is updated on a regular basis and provides more detail on treatment methods presented in this book.

Information regarding most of the treatment methods and on some specific practitioners can also be found on the Web site of the Center for Complementary Medicine at the University of Pittsburgh Medical Center (UPMC):

UPMC Center for Complementary Medicine
5215 Centre Avenue
Pittsburgh, PA 15232
Phone: (412) 623-3023
Web: complementarymedicine.upmc.com

Cardiac Coherence

As the concept of cardiac coherence gains popularity, a number of reputable institutes can help you get started. Check instincttoheal.org for more additions as they become available.

HeartMath Institute
HeartMath LLC
14700 West Park Avenue
Boulder Creek, CA 95006
Phone: (831) 338-8700 or (800) 450-9111
Web: www.heartmath.com

The HeartMath Institute is dedicated to the research and applications of cardiac coherence. You will find information on cardiac coherence and how to obtain the computer program and sensor "Freeze-Framer" described in chapters 3 and 4. This Web site also suggests other books, workshop programs, videos, and brochures.

Berkeley Douglas Ltd. (United Kingdom and Europe)
42 Berkeley Square
London W1J5AW
United Kingdom
Phone: (44) 7000-928-546
E-mail: alanwatkins@berkeleydouglas.com

Under the direction of Alan Watkins, M.D., Ph.D., senior lecturer at the Imperial College of London, Berkeley Douglas offers personal development training and executive coaching in Europe based on the integration of heart coherence with neurophysiology and their use in the development of emotional intelligence.

The Heart of Health, LLC
47–159 Youngs Lane
Indio, CA 92201
Phone: (760) 564-1925
Web: www.theheartofhealth.com
E-mail: roger@tftrx.com

Training sessions and products designed to measure and monitor physiological changes including heart variability and coherence are provided by this company.

Futurehealth Inc.
211 N. Sycamore
Newton, PA 18940
Phone: (215) 504-1700
Web: www.futurehealth.org

Biofeedback and heart rate variability training are taught in this company's "Center for Optimal Living."

Himalayan Institute
R.R. 1, Box 1127
Honesdale, PA 18431
Phone: (570) 253-5551 or (800) 822-4547
Web: www.himalayaninstitute.org

Hatha Yoga is a method that allows participants to experience benefits of "well-being" similar to those brought on by cardiac coherence training. This institute is a leader in the field of yoga and offers weekend and weeklong programs in Hatha Yoga, meditation, stress reduction, and nutrition.

Kripalu Center
P.O. Box 793
West Street, Route 183
Lenox, MA 01240
Phone: (413) 448-3400 or (800) 741-7353
Web: www.kripalu.org
E-mail: request@kripalu.org

The largest center for yoga in the United States with 20 years of experience, Kripalu offers a large number of yoga, self-discovery, and holistic health programs.

Iyengar Yoga Institute of San Francisco
2404 27th Avenue
San Francisco, CA 94116
Phone: (415) 753-0909
Web: www.iyisf.org
E-mail: info@iyisf.org

The Iyengar method of Hatha Yoga is taught at all levels. Information on programs and workshops is also available on this Web site.

Yoga Directory (International)
Web: www.yogadirectory.com

Information on centers and organizations in Europe, Canada, and the United States is listed in this Web site.

Eye Movement Desensitization and Reprocessing (EMDR)

EMDR is a psychotherapy treatment method and therefore should be practiced by a psychiatrist, psychologist, or licensed psychotherapist certified in EMDR. The EMDR Association in the United States and the European EMDR Association in Europe have established strict criteria for the certification process of a clinician. In addition to basic psychotherapy training, the completion of a series of training sessions and supervision by a more experienced therapist are required for certification.

The treatment of a single trauma suffered in everyday life (for example, a fire, an act of aggression, or a serious accident) takes generally fewer than 10 sessions. Sessions usually last up to 90 minutes. Fees vary from $60 to $120. The best way to identify an EMDR-certified psychotherapist in your area is to consult one of the reputable associations below.

EMDR International Association
P.O. Box 141925
Austin, TX 78714
Phone: (512) 451-5200
Web: www.emdria.org

The main objective of this association is to establish and promote the highest standard of excellence by setting up strict criteria for the practice of EMDR.

EMDR Institute (United States)
P.O. Box 51010
Pacific Grove, CA 93950
Phone: (831) 372-3900
Web: www.emdr.com
E-mail: inst@emdr.com

The EMDR Institute provides a directory of certified trained EMDR clinicians in your area. The Web site also compiles information on EMDR research and information about training seminars and workshops.

EMDR Association of Canada
Phone: (306) 665-2788
Web: www.emdrac.ca
E-mail: question@emdrac.ca

The EMDR Association of Canada provides information on practitioners, training seminars, and workshops in Canada.

EMDR Europe Association
Web: www.emdr-europe.net

The European EMDR Association sets standards for the training and practice of EMDR in more than 20 European countries and Israel. It also provides information on practitioners, training seminars, and workshops throughout Europe.

Dawn Simulation

Many different companies manufacture devices to simulate the progressive appearance of dawn prior to a person's awakening. The best ones allow a minimum of 30 minutes of dawn, have an alarm that can be used for the first several nights as a "backup," and are also able to simulate dusk as an aid for falling asleep.

Natural Emporium
14 Forge Court
Madison, WI 53716
Phone: (866) 286-3227
Web: www.naturalemporium.com
E-mail: cs@naturalemporium.com

New Dawn Alarm Clock ($149) uses "smart chip" technology to match an actual morning's sunrise.

Light Therapy Products
6125 Ives Lane North
Plymouth, MN 55442
Phone: (763) 559-1613
Web: www.lighttherapyproducts.com

Products available include SunUp ($156.95) (which is the device that was used in the research experiments of David Avery, M.D., in Seattle), SunRizr ($119.95), Sun Alarm ($78.95), and SunRise Alarm Clock ($99.95).

Pi Square, Inc.
425 Shine Road
Port Ludlow, WA 98635
Phone: (206) 246-1101
Web: www.pi-square.com
E-mail: bps@pi-square.com

Products available include the SunRizr and SunUp.

Outside In Ltd
31 Scotland Rd. Estate
Dry Drayton
Cambridge CB3 8AT
United Kingdom
Phone: + (44)1954-211-953
Web: www.outsidein.co.uk/nac_summ.htm
E-mail: info@putsidein.co.uk

Products available to purchasers in the United Kingdom include three different models of Bodyclocks, ranging in cost from £51 to £85.

Bio-Brite, Inc.
4340 East West Highway, Suite 401S
Bethesda, MD 20814
Phone: (800) 621-LITE or (301) 961-5940

Products available include three different models of SunRise clocks, ranging in cost from approximately $90 to $125.

Acupuncture

This ancient Chinese medicine is gradually gaining a following in the West. Some health insurance carriers now cover acupuncture treatments (although perhaps not for depression). As acupuncture can require a financial investment, be sure to check with your insurance provider—your treatments may qualify for at least partial coverage.

American Academy of Medical Acupuncture
4929 Wilshire Blvd.
Los Angeles, CA 90010
Phone: (323) 937-5514
Web: www.medicalacupuncture.org
E-mail: jdowden@prodigy.net

This association is a professional society for physicians only. A database of physicians practicing acupuncture is available on the Web site.

American Association of Oriental Medicine (AAOM)
5530 Wisconsin Avenue
Chevy Chase, MD 20815
Phone: (301) 941-1064
Web: www.aaom.org
E-mail: info@aaom.org

AAOM was established to develop and administer a national certification to ensure the highest ethical educational standards and a well-regulated profession. Its Web site provides a Directory Search and information on products, resources, education, and state associations.

National Certification Commission for Acupuncture and Oriental Medicine (NCCAOM)
11 Canal Center Plaza, Suite 300
Alexandria, VA 22314
Phone: (703) 548-9004
Web: www.nccaom.org
E-mail: info@nccaom.org

NCCAOM is a nonprofit organization with the main mission to establish and promote standards of competence in acupuncture for the safety of the public. A list of practitioners is available on this Web site.

The Chinese Medicine and Acupuncture Association of Canada
154 Wellington St.
London, Ontario, Canada N6B2K8
Phone: (519) 642-1970
Web: www.cmaac.ca

This is one of the main Canadian associations setting practice standards and providing information on practitioners in Canada.

Omega-3 Fatty Acids

The list of manufacturers and products available is constantly expanding. Instead of providing information that might no longer be valid at the time of the book's publication, I have chosen to list these products on my Web site, which is regularly updated: www.instincttoheal.org.

Many dietary supplements on the market provide a combination of the two essential omega-3 fatty acids, docosahexaenoic acid (DHA) and eicosapentaenoic acid (EPA), contained in fish oils. Standard fish oil usually contains no more than 30 percent omega-3 fatty acids, and a ratio of EPA to DHA of 1.5:1. The best products are those that have the highest concentration of DHA and EPA (more than 90 percent of the oil) in order to minimize the amount of unnecessary calories. Furthermore, some authors, particularly Andrew Stoll, M.D., of Harvard University, recommend the highest EPA amount relative to DHA to maximize the effect on mood elevation and emotional well-being. In the present marketplace, it is possible to find a ratio of EPA to DHA as high as 7:1.

Whatever the product, it is probably best to aim for a daily intake of 1 to 2 grams of EPA (with or without DHA) to be taken before a meal. A high concentration of omega-3 and a high EPA/DHA ratio translate directly into fewer capsules to be taken every day.

Supplements for vegetarians, generally derived from flax seeds, are also available. However, I was not able to find studies documenting the effects of flaxseed products on mood. Based on the amount of the vegetal form of omega-3s contained in flax seeds and flaxseed oil (alpha-linolenic acid) and its rate of conversion into EPA and DHA, it would take approximately 1 to 2 tablespoons of flaxseed oil per day or 4 to 6 tablespoons of whole flax seeds to obtain a mood-enhancing and emotion-balancing effect. (Note that flax seeds should be boiled or lightly broiled and then grinded in a coffee bean grinder in order to minimize the potential for toxicity and to release the maximum amount of alpha-linolenic acid in the body.)

Conflict Management and Emotional Communication

A variety of organizations and practitioners teach emotional communication and conflict management techniques in the family and the corporate environment.

Center for Nonviolent Communication (United States and Europe)
P.O. Box 2662
Sherman, TX 75091
Phone: (903) 893-3886
Web: www.cnvc.org
E-mail: cnvc@cnvc.org

The Center for Nonviolent Communication is a nonprofit organization founded by Marshall B. Rosenberg, Ph.D. (clinical psychologist and author of *Nonviolent Communication: A Language of Compassion*). The center offers worldwide nonviolent communication (NVC) training as well as seminars and workshops. NVC is a method of teaching a person how to express and receive messages from others, even hostile ones, by identifying and recognizing the feelings and needs of others. This empathic understanding is presumed to lead to the reestablishment of a relationship founded on authenticity, clarity, and kindness.

The Gottman Institute
P.O. Box 15644
Seattle, WA 98115
Phone: (206) 523-9042
Web: www.gottman.com
E-mail: gottman@gottman.com

This institute, founded by John Gottman, Ph.D., a researcher and author of *The Relationship Cure* and many other books, and Julie Schwartz Gottman, Ph.D., counsels couples and provides workshops and seminars for both couples and mental health professionals.

International Family Therapy Association
Web: www.ifta-familytherapy.org

IFTA members are therapists, researchers, teachers, and trainers who work with families and couples. Their Web site links to sites related to marriage and family therapy around the world and lists associations, journals, conferences, and referrals.

American Association for Marriage and Family Therapy
112 S. Alfred Street
Alexandria, VA 22314-3061
Phone: (703) 838-9808
Web: www.aamft.org

The Web site provides a directory of family therapists and lists of books, conferences, events, and studies.

Notes

Chapter 1: A New Emotion Medicine

1. Cummings, N. A., and N. Van den Bos, "The Twenty Year Kaiser Permanente Experience with Psychotherapy and Medical Utilization: Implications for National Health Policy and National Health Insurance," *Health Policy Quarterly* 1 (1981): 159–175; Kessler, L. G., P. D. Cleary, et al., "Psychiatric Disorders in Primary Care," *Archives of General Psychiatry* 42 (1985): 583–590; MacFarland, B. H., D. K. Freeborn, et al., "Utilization Patterns Among Long-Term Enrollees in a Prepaid Group Practice Health Maintenance Organization," *Medical Care* 23 (1985): 1121–1233.

2. Grossarth-Maticek, R., and H. J. Eysenck, "Self-Regulation And Mortality From Cancer, Coronary Heart Disease and Other Causes: A Prospective Study," *Personality And Individual Differences* 19 (1995): 781–795.

3. *Pharmacy Times*, "Top ten drugs of 2001," 68 (4) (2002): 10, 12, 15.

4. Antonuccio, D., D. D. Burns, et al., "Antidepressants: A Triumph of Marketing Over Science?" *Prevention & Treatment* 5, Article 25, posted July 15, 2002.

5. Langer, G., "Use of Antidepressants is a Long-term Practice," www.abcnews.com (2000).

6. Kessler, R., J. Soukup, et al., "The Use of Complementary and Alternative Therapies to Treat Anxiety and Depression in the United States," *American Journal of Psychiatry* 158 (2001): 289–294.

7. Gabbard, G. O., J. G. Gunderson, et al., "The Place of Psychoanalytic Treatments within Psychiatry," *Archives of General Psychiatry* 59 (2002): 505–510.

8. Kramer, P., *Listening to Prozac* (New York: Viking, 1993).

9. Flint, A., and S. Rifat, "Recurrence of First-Episode Geriatric Depression after Discontinuation of Maintenance Antidepressants," *American Journal of Psychiatry* 156 (1999): 943–945; Frank, E., D. Kupfer, et al., "Early Recurrence in Unipolar Depression," *Archives of General Psychiatry* 46, no. 5 (1989): 397–400; G. Goodwin, "Recurrence of Mania after Lithium Withdrawal: Implications for the Use of Lithium in the Treatment of Bipolar Affective Disorder," *British Journal of Psychiatry* 164 (1994): 149–152; J. Littrell, "Relationship Between Time Since Reuptake-blocker Antidepressant Discontinuation and Relapse," *Experimental & Clinical Psychopharmacology* 2 (1994): 82–94; E. Peselow, D. Dunner, et al., "The Prophylactic Efficacy of Tricyclic Antidepressants: A Five Year Follow-up," *Progress in Neuro-Psychopharmacology & Biological Psychiatry* 15, no.1 (1991): 71–82; Baldessarini, R., and A. Viguera, "Neuroleptic withdrawal in schizophrenic patients," *Archives of General Psychiatry* 52, no. 3 (1995): 189–192.

10. Viguera, A., R. Baldessarini, et al., "Discontinuing Antidepressant Treatment in Major Depression," *Harvard Review of Psychiatry* 5, no. 6 (1998): 293–306.

Chapter 2: Discontent in Neurobiology

1. Mayer, J. D., P. Salovey, A. Capuso, "Models of Emotional Intelligence," in Steinberg, R. J. (ed.), *Handbook of Intelligence* (Cambridge: Cambridge University Press, 2000).

2. Goleman, D., *Emotional Intelligence* (New York: Bantam Books, 1995).

3. Mayer, et al., *Handbook of Intelligence*, 396–420.

4. Vaillant, G., *Adaptation to Life* (Boston: Harvard University Press, 1995).

5. Felsman, J. K., and G. Vaillant, "Resilient Children as Adults: A 40-Year Study," in *The Invulnerable Child*, eds. E. J. Anderson and B. J. Cohler (New York: Guilford Press, 1987).

6. Broca, P., "Anatomie Comparée des Circonvolutions Cérébrales. Le Grand Lobe Limbique et la Scissure Limbique dans la Série des Ammifières," *Revue Anthropologique* 2 (1878): 385–498.

7. Servan-Schreiber, D., W. M. Perlstein, et al., "Selective Pharmacological Activation of Limbic Structures in Human Volunteers: A Positron Emission Tomography Study," *Journal of Neuropsychiatry and Clinical Neurosciences* 10 (1998): 148–159.

8. LeDoux, J. E., *The Emotional Brain: The Mysterious Underpinnings of Emotional Life* (New York: Simon & Schuster, 1996).

9. Levitt, P, "A monoclonal antibody to limbic system neurons," *Science* 223 (1984): 299–301.

10. Damasio, A., *The Feeling of What Happens* (San Diego: Harcourt, 1990). In his most recent book, Damasio explores the consequences of this notion further, and attributes the discovery of the connection between emotions and physiological reactions in the body to the great 17th-century philosopher Benedict (Baruch) Spinoza; Damasio, A., *Looking for Spinoza: Joy, Sorrow and the Feeling Brain* (San Diego: Harcourt, 2003).

11. Mehler, J., G. Lambertz, et al., "Discrimination de la Langue Maternelle par le Nouveau-né," *Comptes Rendus de l'Académie des Sciences* 303 (1986): 637–640.

12. Arnsten, A. F., and P. S. Goldman-Rakic, "Noise Stress Impairs Prefrontal Cortical Cognitive Function in Monkeys: Evidence for a Hyperdopaminergic Mechanism," *Archives of General Psychiatry* 55, no. 4 (1998): 362–368.

13. Regier, D. A., and Robins, L. N., *Psychiatric Disorders in America: The Epidemiology Catchment Area Study* (New York: Free Press, 1991).

14. Ochsner, K. N., S. A. Bunge, et al., "An MRI study of the cognitive regulation of emotion," *Journal of Cognitive Neuroscience* (2002). See also the theory of Drevets and Raichle, who describe the relationship of reciprocal inhibition between the cognitive and emotional brains and the confirmation of that theory in a recent study at Duke University with MRI by Yamasaki and LaBar. Drevets, W. C., and M. E. Raichle, "Reciprocal Suppression of Regional Cerebral Blood Flow During Emotional Versus Higher Cognitive Processes: Implications for Interactions between Emotion and Cognition," *Cognition and Emotion* 12 (1998): 353–385; Yamasaki, H., K. S. LaBar, et al., "Dissociable prefrontal brain systems for attention and emotion," *Proceedings of the National Academy of Sciences* 99, no. 17 (2002): 11447–11451.

15. Macmillan, M. B. (1986), "A wonderful journey through skull and brains: The travels of Mr. Gage's tamping iron," *Brain and Cognition*, no. 5 (1986): 67–107.

16. Damasio, H., T. Brabowski, et al., "The Return of Phineas Gage: Clues about the Brain from the Skull of a Famous Patient," *Science* 264 (1994): 1102–1105.

17. Eslinger, P. J., and A. R. Damasio, "Severe Disturbance of Higher Cognition after Bilateral Frontal Lobe Ablation: Patient EVR," *Neurology* 35 (1985): 1731–1741.

18. Levenson, R., et al., "The Influence of Age and Gender on Affect, Physiology, and their Interrelations: A Study of Long-Term Marriages," *Journal of Personality and Social Psychology* 67 (1994).

19. Csikszentmihalyi, M., *Flow: The Psychology of Optimal Experience* (New York: Harper & Row, 1990).

Chapter 3: The Heart and Its Reasons

1. Harrer, G., and H. Harrer, "Music, Emotion and Autonomic Function," *Music and the Brain*, M. Critchley and R. A. Hanson eds. (London: William Heinemann Medical, 1977) 202–215.

2. Grossarth-Maticek, R., and H. J. Eysenck, "Self-regulation and Mortality from Cancer, Coronary Heart Disease and Other Causes: A Prospective Study," *Personality and Individual Differences* 19, no. 6 (1995): 781–795; Linden, W., C. Stossel, et al., "Psychosocial Interventions for Patients with Coronary Artery Disease: A Meta-Analysis," *Archives of Internal Medicine* 156, no. 7 (1996): 745–752; Ornish, D., L. Scherwitz, et al., "Intensive Lifestyle Changes for Reversal of Coronary Heart Disease," *Journal of the American Medical Association* 280, no. 23 (1998): 2001–2007.

3. Frasure-Smith, N., F. Lesperance, et al., "Depression and 18-Month Prognosis after Myocardial Infarction," *Circulation* 91, no. 4 (1995): 999–1005; Glassman, A., and P. Shapiro, "Depression and the Course of Coronary Artery Disease," *American Journal of Psychiatry* 155 (1998): 4–10.

4. Armour, J. A., and J. Ardell, *Neurocardiology* (New York: Oxford University Press, 1994); Samuels, M., "Voodoo Death Revisited: The Modern Lessons of Neurocardiology," Grand Rounds, Department of Medicine, University of Pittsburgh Medical Center, Presbyterian/ Shadyside Hospital, 2001.

5. Armour, J. A., ed., "Anatomy and Function of the Intrathoracic Neurons Regulating the Mammalian Heart," *Reflex Control of the*

Circulation (Boca Raton, FL: CRC Press, 1991); Gershon, M. D., "The Enteric Nervous System: A Second Brain," *Hospital Practice* (Office Edition) 34, no. 7 (1999): 31–32, 35–38, 41–42 passim.

6. Carter, C. S., "Neuroendocrine Perspectives on Social Attachment and Love," *Psychoneuroendocrinology* 23 (1998): 779–818; Uvnas-Moberg, K., "Oxytocin May Mediate the Benefits of Positive Social Interaction and Emotions," *Psychoneuroendocrinology* 23 (1998): 819–835. The Quebec researchers, Cantin and Genest, after discovering the ANF (atrial natriuretic factor), were among the first to describe the heart as an actual hormonal gland in their article: Cantin, M., and J. Genest, "The heart as an endocrine gland," *Clinical and Investigative Medicine* 9, no. 4 (1986): 319–327.

7. Stroink, G., "Principles of Cardiomagnetism," *Advances in Biomagnetism*, S. J. Williamson et al. eds. (New York: Plenum Press, 1989) 47–57.

8. Coplan, J. D., L. A. Papp, et al., "Amelioration of Mitral Valve Prolapse after Treatment for Panic Disorder," *American Journal of Psychiatry* 149, no.11 (1992): 1587–1588.

9. Gahery, Y., and D. Vigier, "Inhibitory Effects in the Cuneate Nucleus Produced by Vago-Aortic Afferent Fibers," *Brain Research* 75 (1974): 241–246.

10. Akselrod, S., D. Gordon, et al., "Power Spectrum Analysis of Heart Rate Fluctuation: A Quantitative Probe of Beat-to-Beat Cardiovascular Control," *Science* 213 (1981): 220–222.

11. Umetani, K., D. Singer, et al., "Twenty-Four Hours Time Domain Heart Rate Variability and Heart Rate: Relations to Age and Gender over Nine Decades," *Journal of the American College of Cardiology* 31, no. 3 (1999): 593–601.

12. Tsuji, H., F. Venditti, et al., "Reduced Heart Rate Variability and Mortality Risk in an Elderly Cohort. The Framingham Heart Study," *Circulation* 90, no. 2 (1994): 878–883; Dekker, J., E. Schouten, et al., "Heart Rate Variability from Short Term Electrocardiographic Recordings Predicts Mortality from All Causes in Middle-Aged and Elderly

Men. The Zutphen Study," *American Journal of Epidemiology* 145, no.10 (1997): 899–908; La Rovere, M., J. T. Bigger, et al., "Baroreflex Sensitivity and Heart-Rate Variability in Prediction of Total Cardiac Mortality after Myocardial Infarction," *The Lancet* 351 (1998): 478–484.

13. Carney, R. M., M. W. Rich, et al., "The Relationship between Heart Rate, Heart Rate Variability, and Depression in Patients with Coronary Artery Disease," *Journal of Psychosomatic Research* 32 (1988): 159–164; Rechlin, T., M. Weis, et al., "Are Affective Disorders Associated with Alterations of Heart Rate Variability?" *Journal of Affective Disorders* 32, no. 4 (1994): 271–275; Krittayaphong, R., W. Cascio, et al., "Heart rate variability in patients with coronary artery disease: differences in patients with higher and lower depression scores," *Psychosomatic Medicine* 59, no. 3 (1997): 231–235; Stys, A., and T. Stys, "Current clinical applications of heart rate variability," *Clinical Cardiology* 21 (1998): 719–724; Carney, R., K. Freedland, et al., "Change in Heart Rate Variability During Treatment for Depression in Patients with Coronary Heart Disease," *American Psychosomatic Society* 62, no. 5 (2000): 639–647; Luskin, F., M. Reitz, et al., "A Controlled Pilot Study of Stress Management Training in Elderly Patients with Congestive Heart Failure," *Preventive Cardiology* 5, no. 4 (2002): 168–172.

14. McCraty, R., M. Atkinson, et al., "The Effects of Emotions on Short-Term Power Spectrum Analysis and Heart Rate Variability," *The American Journal of Cardiology* 76, no.14 (1995): 1089–1093.

15. Barrios-Choplin, B., R. McCraty, et al., "An Inner Quality Approach to Reducing Stress and Improving Physical and Emotional Well-Being at Work," *Stress Medicine* 13, no. 3 (1997): 193–201.

16. Watkins, A. D., "Corporate Training In Heart Rate Variability: 6 Weeks and 6 Months Follow-Up Studies," Hunter-Kane, London (2002).

17. Katz, L. F., and J. M. Gottman, "Buffering Children from Marital Conflict and Dissolution," *Journal of Clinical Child Psychology* 26 (1997): 157–171.

Chapter 4: Living with Heart Coherence

1. McCraty, R., ed., *Science of the Heart: Exploring the Role of the Heart in Human Performance* (Boulder Creek, CA: Institute of HeartMath, 2001).

2. McCraty, R., M. Atkinson, et al., "The Effects of Emotions on Short-Term Power Spectrum Analysis and Heart Rate Variability," *The American Journal of Cardiology* 76, no. 14 (1995): 1089–1093.

3. Luskin, F., M. Reitz, et al., "A Controlled Pilot Study of Stress Management Training in Elderly Patients with Congestive Heart Failure," *Preventive Cardiology* 5, no. 4 (2002): 168–172.

4. Barrios-Choplin, B., R. McCraty, et al., "An Inner Quality Approach to Reducing Stress and Improving Physical and Emotional Well-Being at Work," *Stress Medicine* 13, no. 3 (1997): 193–201.

5. Baulieu, E., G. Thomas, et al., "Dehydroepiandrosterone (DHEA), DHEA Sulfate, and Aging: Contribution of the DHEA Study to a Sociobiomedical Issue," *Proceedings of the National Academy of Science* 97, no. 8 (2000): 4279–4284.

6. Kirschbaum, C., O. Wolf, et al., "Stress and Treatment-Induced Elevation of Cortisol Levels Associated with Impaired Declarative Memory in Healthy Adults," *Life Sciences* 58, no. 17 (1996): 1475–1483; Bremner, J. D., "Does Stress Damage the Brain?" *Society of Biological Psychiatry* 45 (1999): 797–805; McEwen, B., *The End of Stress as We Know It* (Washington, DC: National Academic Press, 2002).

7. McCraty, R., B. Barrios-Choplin, et al., "The Impact of a New Emotional Self-Management Program on Stress, Emotions, Heart Rate Variability, DHEA and Cortisol," *Integrative Physiological and Behavioral Science* 33, no. 2 (1998): 151–170.

8. Rein, G., R. McCraty, et al., "Effects of Positive and Negative Emotions on Salivary IgA," *Journal for the Advancement of Medicine* 8, no. 2 (1995): 87–105.

9. Cohen, S., D. A. Tyrrell, et al., "Psychological Stress and Susceptibility to the Common Cold," *New England Journal of Medicine* 325, no. 9 (1991): 606–612.

10. McCraty, R., ed., *Science of the Heart: Exploring the Role of the Heart in Human Performance* (Boulder Creek, CA: Institute of HeartMath, 2001).

11. *Ibid.*

Chapter 5: Eye Movement Desensitization and Reprocessing

1. Rauch, S. L., Van der Kolk et al., "A Symptom Provocation Study of Posttraumatic Stress Disorder Using Positron Emission Tomography and Script-Driven Imagery," *Archives of General Psychiatry* 53 (1996): 380–387. There have been several other brain imaging studies of PTSD since then that have pointed to a number of other brain regions possibly being involved in PTSD. This remains an active area of research with the usual disagreements and controversies over the interpretation of findings. I chose to illustrate the neural correlates of PTSD with this older study because it captures so well—at the neurological level—the essence of what we see as clinicians: strong emotions, vivid visual images, and impaired verbal expression.

2. Breslau, N., R. C. Kessler, et al., "Trauma and Posttraumatic Stress Disorder in the Community: The 1996 Detroit Area Survey of Trauma," *Archives of General Psychiatry* 55 (1998): 626–632.

3. Shapiro, F., *EMDR Treatment: Overview and Integration. EMDR as an Integrative Psychotherapy Approach* (Washington, DC: American Psychological Association, 2002).

4. LeDoux, J. E., "Brain Mechanisms of Emotions and Emotional Learning," *Current Opinion in Neurobiology* 2 (1992): 191–197.

5. Pavlov, I. P., *Conditioned Reflexes* (London: Oxford University Press, 1927).

6. Quirk, G. I., "Memory for Extinction of Conditioned Fear is Long-Lasting and Persists Following Spontaneous Recovery," *Learning and Memory* 9, no. 6 (2002): 402–407; Morgan, M. A., L. M. Romanski, et al. "Extinction of Emotional Learning: Contribution of Medial Prefrontal Cortex," *Neuroscience Letters* 163, no. 1 (1993): 109–113.

7. LeDoux, J. E., L. Romanski, et al., "Indelibility of Subcortical Emotional Memories," *Journal of Cognitive Neuroscience* 1 (1989): 238–243. LeDoux, J. E., *The Emotional Brain: The Mysterious Underpinnings of Emotional Life* (New York: Simon & Schuster, 1996).

8. See the neural network of this phenomenon developed by Jorge Armony in LeDoux's lab in collaboration with my own laboratory at the University of Pittsburgh: Armony, J., D. Servan-Schreiber, et al., "Computational Modeling of Emotion: Explorations Through the Anatomy and Physiology of Fear Conditioning," *Trends in Cognitive Sciences* 1, no. 1 (1997): 28–34.

9. Solomon, S., E. T. Gerrity, et al., "Efficacy of Treatments for Posttraumatic Stress Disorder," *Journal of the American Medical Association* 268 (1992): 633–638.

10. Wilson, S., L. Becker, et al., "Eye Movement Desensitization and Reprocessing (EMDR) Treatment for Psychologically Traumatized Individuals," *Journal of Consulting and Clinical Psychology* 63 (1995): 928–937; Wilson, S., L. Becker, et al., "Fifteen-Month Follow-Up of Eye Movement Desensitization and Reprocessing (EMDR) Treatment for Posttraumatic Stress Disorder and Psychological Trauma," *Journal of Consulting and Clinical Psychology* 65 (1997): 1047–1056.

11. Antibiotics are successful in 90 percent of outpatient cases of pneumonia but only 80 percent of patients who require hospitalization. Those cases, of course, are more serious. Fine, M., R. Stone, et al., "Processes and Outcomes of Care for Patients with Community-Acquired Pneumonia," *Archives of Internal Medicine* 159 (1999): 970–980.

12. Shapiro, F., *Eye Movement Desensitization and Reprocessing: Basic Principles, Protocols and Procedures*, 2nd ed. (New York: Guilford, 2001); Stickgold, R., "EMDR: A Putative Neurobiological Mechanism," *Journal of Clinical Psychology* 58 (2002): 61–75.

13. Cyrulnik, B., *Les Vilains Petits Canards* (Paris: Odile Jacob, 2001).

14. Van Der Kolk, B., "Beyond the Talking Cure: Somatic Experience and the Subcortical Imprints in the Treatment of Trauma," in *EMDR as an Integrative Psychotherapy Approach*, F. Shapiro, ed. (Wash-

ington, DC: American Psychological Association, 2002); Shapiro, F., *Eye Movement Desensitization and Reprocessing: Basic Principles, Protocols and Procedures* (New York: Guilford, 2001).

15. Rumelhart, D. E., and J. L. McClelland, *Parallel Distributed Processing: Explorations in the Microstructure of Cognition* (Cambridge, MA: MIT Press, 1986); Edelman, G. N., *Neural Darwinism: The Theory of Neuronal Group Selection* (New York: Perseus Publishing, 1987).

16. The title of one of Bessel van der Kolk's early papers on this issue used a quote from one of his multiply traumatized patients, "The Body Keeps the Score . . ." van der Kolk, B. A., "The Body Keeps the Score: Memory and the Evolving Psychobiology of Posttraumatic Stress," *Harvard Review of Psychiatry* 1 (1994): 253–265.

Chapter 6: EMDR in Action

1. Kübler-Ross, E., *On Death and Dying* (New York: Touchstone, 1969).

2. Chemtob, C. M., J. Nakashima, et al., "Brief Treatment for Elementary School Children with Disaster-Related Post-Traumatic Stress Disorder: A Field Study," *Journal of Clinical Psychology* 58 (2002): 99–112.

3. Van Etten, M. L., and S. Taylor, "Comparative Efficacy of Treatments for Post-Traumatic Stress Disorder: A Meta-Analysis," *Clinical Psychology & Psychotherapy* 5 (1998): 126–144; Spector, J., and J. Read, "The Current Status of Eye Movement Desensitization and Reprocessing (EMDR)," *Clinical Psychology & Psychotherapy* 6 (1999): 165–174; Sack, M., W. Lempa, et al., "Study Quality and Effect-Sizes: A Meta-Analysis of EMDR-Treatment for Post-Traumatic Stress Disorder," *Psychotherapie, Psychosomatik, Medizinische Psychologie* 51, no. 9–10 (2001): 350–355; Maxfield, L., and L. A. Hyer, "The Relationship Between Efficacy and Methodology in Studies Investigating EMDR Treatment of PTSD," *Journal of Clinical Psychology* 58 (2002): 23–41.

4. Herbert, J., S. Lilienfeld, et al., "Science and Pseudoscience in the Development of Eye Movement Desensitization and Reprocessing: Implications for Clinical Psychology," *Clinical Psychology Review* 20 (2000): 945–971. A detailed reply to this criticism was published by two American psychoanalysts in 2002: Perkins, B. R., and C. C. Rouanzoin, "A Critical Evaluation of Current Views Regarding Eye Movement Desensitization and Reprocessing (EMDR): Clarifying Points of Confusion," *Journal of Clinical Psychology* 58 (2002): 77–97.

5. Stickgold, R., J. A. Hobson, et al., "Sleep, Learning, and Dreams: Off-Line Memory Reprocessing," *Science* (2001): 1052–1057.

6. Stickgold, R.,"EMDR: A Putative Neurobiological Mechanism," *Journal of Clinical Psychology* 58 (2002): 61–75.

7. Wilson, D., S. M. Silver, et al., "Eye Movement Desensitization and Reprocessing: Effectiveness and Autonomic Correlates," *Journal of Behavior Therapy and Experimental Psychiatry* 27 (1996).

8. Pessah, M. A., and H. P. Roffwarg, "Spontaneous Middle Ear Muscle Activity in Man: A Rapid Eye Movement Sleep Phenomenon," *Science* 178 (1972): 773–776; Benson, K., and V. P. Zarcone, "Phasic Events of REM Sleep: Phenomenology of Middle Ear Muscle Activity and Periorbital Integrated Potentials in the Same Normal Population," *Sleep* 2, no. 2 (1979): 199–213.

9. Servan-Schreiber, D.,"Eye Movement Desensitization and Reprocessing: Is Psychiatry Missing the Point?" *Psychiatric Times* 17, no. 7 (2000): 36–40.

10. Chambless, D., M. Baker, et al., "Update on Empirically Validated Therapies, II," *The Clinical Psychologist* 51, no. 1 (1998): 3–16.

11. Chemtob, C. M., D. Tolin, et al., "Eye Movement Desensitization and Reprocessing (EMDR)," in *Effective Treatments for PTSD: Practice Guidelines from the International Society for Traumatic Stress Studies*, E. A. Foa, T. M. Keane, and M. J. Friedman, eds. (New York: Guilford Press, 2000): 139–155, 333–335.

12. United Kingdom Department of Health, "The Evidence Based Clinical Practice Guideline" (2001).

13. Bleich, A., J. Berstein, et. al., "Guidelines for the Assessment and Professional Intervention with Terror Victims in the Hospital and in the Community," a position paper of the National Council for Mental Health, Ministry of Health, Israel (2002).

14. CREST, "The Management of Posttraumatic Stress Disorder in Adults" (Belfast, Ireland, Clinical Resource Efficiency Support Team of the Northern Ireland Department of Health, Social Services and Public Safety, 2003).

15. Kirsch, I., A. Scoboria, et al., "Antidepressants and Placebos: Secrets, Revelations, and Unanswered Questions," *Prevention & Treatment* (2002); Thase, M. E., "Antidepressant Effects: The Suit May Be Small, but the Fabric is Real," Article 32, *Prevention & Treatment* (2002); Khan, A., R. Leventhal, et al., "Severity of Depression and Response to Antidepressants and Placebo: An Analysis of the Food and Drug Administration Database," *Journal of Clinical Psychopharmacology* 22, no. 1 (2002): 50–54.

16. Yehuda, R., A. C. McFarlane, et al., "Predicting the Development of Post-Traumatic Stress Disorder from the Acute Response to a Traumatic Event," *Biological Psychiatry* 44 (1998): 1305–1313.

Chapter 7: The Energy of Light

1. Cook, F. A., "Medical Observations Among the Esquimaux," *New York Journal of Gynecology and Obstetrics* 4 (1894): 282–296, cited in Rosenthal, N. E., *Winter Blues: Seasonal Affective Disorder—What It Is and How to Overcome It* (New York: Guilford Press, 1998).

2. Haggarty, J. M., Z. Cernovsh et al., "The Limited Influence of Latitude on Rates of Seasonal Affective Disorder," *Journal of Nervous and Mental Disease* 189 (2001): 482–484.

3. Avery, D. H., D. N. Eder, et al., "Dawn Simulation and Bright

Light in the Treatment of SAD: A Controlled Study," *Biological Psychiatry* 50, no. 3 (2001): 205–216.

4. Personal communication of e-mail sent Don Romero of Pi-Square, Inc., Seattle, Washington.

5. Parry, B., S. Berga, et al., "Melatonin and Phototherapy in Premenstrual Depression," *Progress in Clinical & Biological Research* 341 B (1990): 35–43; Lam, R. W., E. M. Goldner, et al., "A Controlled Study of Light Therapy for Bulimia Nervosa," *American Journal of Psychiatry* 151, no. 5 (1994): 744–750; Satlin, A., L. Volicer, et al., "Bright Light Treatment of Behavioral and Sleep Disturbances in Patients with Alzheimer's Disease," *Amercian Journal of Psychiatry* 149, no. 8 (1992): 1028–1032; Levitt, A., R. Joffe, et al., "Bright Light Augmentation in Antidepressant Nonresponders," *Journal of Clinical Psychiatry* 52, no. 8 (1991): 336–337.

6. In-Young, Y., D. Kripke, et al., "Luteinizing Hormone Following Light Exposure in Healthy Young Men," *Neuroscience Letters* 341, no. 1 (2003): 25–28.

Chapter 8: The Power of Qi

1. Soulie de Morant, G. I., *L'Acupuncture Chinoise* (Paris: Maloine Éditeurs, 1972).

2. As analyses of all the clinical studies registered by the American Food and Drug Adminstration suggest: Kirsch, I., A. Scoboria, et al., "Antidepressants and Placebos: Secrets, Revelations, and Unanswered Questions," *Prevention & Treatment* (2002); Thase, M. E., "Antidepressant Effects: The Suit May Be Small, but the Fabric is Real," *Prevention & Treatment* Article 32 (2002); Khan, A., R. Leventhal, et al., "Severity of Depression and Response to Antidepressants and Placebo: An Analysis of the Food and Drug Administration Database," *Journal of Clinical Psychopharmacology* 22, no. 1 (2002): 50–54.

3. British Medical Association, Board of Sciences, *Acupuncture: Efficacy, Safety and Practice* (London: Harwood Academic, 2000).

4. Ulett, G. A., S. Han, et al., "Electroacupuncture: Mechanisms and Clinical Applications," *Biological Psychiatry* 44 (1998): 129–138.

5. Hechun, L., J. Yunkui, et al., "Electroacupuncture vs. Amitriptyline in the Treatment of Depressive States," *Journal of Traditional Chinese Medicine* (1985): 3–8; Han, J.-S., "Electroacupuncture: An Alternative to Antidepressants for Treating Affective Diseases?" *Journal of Neuroscience* 29 (1986): 79–92; Polyakov, S. E., "Acupuncture in the Treatment of Endogenous Depression," *Soviet Neurology and Psychiatry* 21 (1988): 36–44; Thomas, M., S. V. Eriksson, et al., "A Comparative Study of Diazepam and Acupuncture in Patients with Osteoarthritis Pain: A Placebo Controlled Study," *American Journal of Chinese Medicine* 2, no. XIX (1991): 95–100; Jin, H., L. Zhou, et al., "The Inhibition by Electrical Acupuncture on Gastric Acid Secretion is Mediated Via Endorphin and Somatostating in Dogs," *Clinical Research* 40 (1992): 167A; Li, Y., G. Tougas, et al., "The Effect of Acupuncture on Gastrointestinal Function and Disorders," *American Journal of Gastroenterology* 87 (1992): 1372–1381; He, D., J. Berg, et al., "Effects of Acupuncture on Smoking Cessation or Reduction for Motivated Smokers," *Preventive Medicine* 26 (1997): 208–214; Cardini, F. W., Huang, "Moxibustion for Correction of Breech Presentation," *Journal of the American Medical Association* 280, no. 18 (1998): 1580–1584; Montakab, H., "Akupunktur und Schlaflosigkeit [Acupuncture and insomnia]," *Forschende Komplementarmedizin* 6 (Supplement 1) (1999): 29–31; Timofeev, M. F., "Effects of Acupuncture and an Agonist of Opiate Receptors on Heroin Dependent Patients," *American Journal of Chinese Medicine* 27, no. 2 (1999): 143–148; Wang, S.-M., and Z. N. Kain, "Auricular Acupuncture: A Potential Treatment for Anxiety," *Anesthesia and Analgesia* 92 (2001): 548–553; Paulus, W. E., M. Zhang, et al., "Influence of Acupuncture on the Pregnancy Rate in Pa-

tients Who Undergo Assisted Reproduction Therapy," *Fertility and Sterility* 77, no. 4 (2002): 721–724.

6. Cho, Z. H., S. C. Chung, et al., "New Findings of the Correlation Between Acupoints and Corresponding Brain Cortices Using Functional MRI," *Proceedings of the National Academy of Sciences* 95 (1998): 2670–2673.

7. Han, *op. cit.*; Luo, H. C., Y. K. Jia, et al., "Electroacupuncture vs. Amitriptyline in the Treatment of Depressive States," *Journal of Traditional Chinese Medicine* 5 (1985): 3–8; Lou, H. C., Y. Jia, et al., "Electro-acupuncture in the Treatment of Depressive Psychosis," *International Journal fo Clinical Acupuncture* 1 (1990): 7–13; Luo, H. C., Y. C. Shen, et al., "A Comparative Study of the Treatment of Depression by Electroacupuncture and Amitriptyline," *Acupuncture* 1 (Huntington, NY: 1990) 20–26.

8. Wang, *op. cit.* (2001).

9. Hui, K., J. Liu, et al., "Acupuncture Modulates the Limbic System and Subcortical Gray Structures of the Human Brain: Evidence from MRI Studies in Normal Subjects," *Human Brain Mapping* 9 (2000): 13–25.

10. Chen, L., J. Tang, et al., "The Effect of Location of Transcutaneous Electrical Nerve Stimulation on Postoperative Opioid Analgesic Requirement: Acupoint Versus Nonacupoint Stimulation," *Anesth Analg* 87 (1998): 1129–1134; Lao, L., S. Bergman, et al., "Evaluation of Acupuncture for Pain Control after Oral Surgery: A Placebo-Controlled Trial," *Archives of Otolaryngology—Head and Neck Surgery* 125 (1999): 567–572.

11. Haker, E., H. Egekvist, et al., "Effect of DSensory Stimulation Cacupuncture) on sympathetic and parasympathetic activites in healthy subjects," *Journal of the Autonomic Nervous System* 79, no. 1 (2000): 52–59.

12. Pert, C. B., H. E. Dreher, et al., "The Psychosomatic Network: Foundations of Mind-Body Medicine," *Alternative Therapies in Health and Medicine* 4, no. 4 (1998): 30–41.

Chapter 9: The Revolution in Nutrition

1. Bågedahl-Strindlund, M., and K. Monsen Börjesson, "Postnatal Depression: A Hidden Illness," *Acta Psychiatrica Scandinavica* 98 (1998): 272–275.

2. Hibbeln, J. R., "Long-Chain Polyunsaturated Fatty Acids in Depression and Related Conditions," *Phospholipid spectrum disorder*, M. Peet, I. Glen, and D. Horrobin (Lancashire, U.K.: Marius Press, 1999), 195–210.

3. Hornstra, G., M. Al, et al., "Essential Fatty Acids in Pregnancy and Early Human Development," *European Journal of Obstetrics, Gynecology, and Reproductive Biology* 61, no. 1 (1995): 57–62; Al, M., A. C. van Houwelingen, et al., "Long-Chain Polyunsaturated Fatty Acids, Pregnancy, And Pregnancy Outcome," *American Journal of Clinical Nutrition* 71 (2000): 285S–291S.

4. Hibbeln, J., "Fish Consumption and Major Depression," *The Lancet* 351 (1998): 1213.

5. Barton, P. G., and F. D. Gunstone, "Hydrocarbon Chain Packing and Molecular Motion in Phospholipid Bilayers Formed from Unsaturated Lecithin," *Journal of Biological Chemistry* 250 (1975): 4470–4476; Sperling, R. I., A. I. Benincaso, et al., "Dietary Omega-3 Polyunsaturated Fatty Acids Inhibit Phosphoinositide Formation and Chemotaxis in Neutrophils," *Journal of Clinical Investigation* 91 (1993): 651–660.

6. Bourre, J. M., M. Bonneil, et al., "Function of Dietary Polyunsaturated Fatty Acids in the Nervous System," *Prostaglandins Leukotrienes & Essential Fatty Acids* 48, no. 1 (1993): 5–15.

7. Frances, H., P. Drai, et al., "Nutritional (n-3) Polyunsaturated Fatty Acids Influence the Behavioral Responses to Positive Events in Mice," *Neuroscience Letters* 285, no. 3 (2000): 223–227.

8. Bang, H. O., J. Dyerberg, et al., "The Composition of Foods Consumed by Greenland Eskimos," *Acta Medica Scandinavica* 200 (1976): 69–73.

9. This concerns primarily dopamine, the neurotransmitter responsible for the euphoria and surge of energy associated with cocaine and amphetamines. Chalon, S., S. Delion-Vancassel, et al., "Dietary Fish Oil Affects Monoaminergic Neurotransmission and Behavior in Rats," *Journal of Nutrition* 128 (1998): 2512–2519.

10. Olsen, S. F., and N. J. Secher, "Low Consumption of Seafood in Early Pregnancy as a Risk Factor for Preterm Delivery: Prospective Cohort Study," *British Medical Journal* 324 (2002): 447–451.

11. Naturally, the difference in IQ may be explained by other factors as well, such as a better emotional connection with the infants among mothers who breastfed for a longer period, etcetera. However, there is a consensus among researchers about the importance of an adequate supply of omega-3 fatty acids for brain development in the newborn. Mortensen, E. L., K. F. Michaelsen, et al., "The Association Between Duration of Breastfeeding and Adult Intelligence," *Journal of the American Medical Association* 287 (2002): 2365–2371.

12. Hibbeln, J., "Seafood consumption, The DHA Content of Mothers' Milk and Prevalence Rates of Postpartum Depression: A Cross-National, Ecological Analysis," *Journal of Affective Disorders* 69 (2002): 15–29.

13. Stoll, A. L., W. E. Severus, et al., "Omega 3 Fatty Acids in Bipolar Disorder: A Preliminary Double-Blind, Placebo-Controlled Trial," *Archives of General Psychiatry* 56 (1999): 407–412.

14. Stoll, A. L., *The Omega-3 Connection: The Groundbreaking Omega-3 Antidepression Diet and Brain Program* (New York: Simon & Schuster, 2001).

15. A preliminary study of the effects of an esterified extract of fish oil on stage III of Huntington's disease—the most advanced stage of the illness—shows an improvement of symptoms over a few months compared to the group taking an olive oil placebo. It also shows a rebuilding of cortical tissue as opposed to the steady withering of cortex in the control group. This suggests an inversion of the pathological processes in the brain underlying the illness.

16. Zanarini, M., and F. R. Frankenburg, "Omega-3 Fatty Acid Treatment of Women with Borderline Personality Disorder: A Double-Blind, Placebo-Controlled Pilot Study," *American Journal of Psychiatry* 160 (2003): 167–169.

17. Maes, M., R. Smith, et al., "Fatty Acid Composition in Major Depression: Decreased w3 Fractions in Cholesteryl Esters And Increased C20:4 Omega 6/C20:5 Omega 3 Ratio in Cholesteryl Esters and Phospholipids," *Journal of Affective Disorders* 38 (1996): 35–46; Peet, M., B. Murphy, et al.,"Depletion of Omega-3 Fatty Acid Levels in Red Blood Cell Membranes of Depressive Patient," *Biological Psychiatry* 43, no. 5 (1998): 315–319.

18. Adams, P. B., S. Lawson, et al., "Arachidonic Acid to Eicosapentanoic Acid Ratio in Blood Correlates Positively with Clinical Symptoms of Depression," *Lipids* 31 (1996): S157–S161.

19. Edwards, R., M. Peet, et al., "Omega-3 Polyunsaturated Fatty Acid Levels in the Diet and in Red Blood Cell Membranes of Depressed Patients," *Journal of Affective Disorders* 48, no. 2–3 (1998): 149–155.

20. Tanskanen, A., J. Hibbeln, et al., "Fish Consumption, Depression, and Suicidality in a General Population," *Archives of General Psychiatry* 58 (2001): 512–513.

21. Tiemeier, H., H. van Tuijl, et al., "Plasma Fatty Acid Composition and Depression Are Associated in the Elderly: The Rotterdam Study," *American Journal of Clinical Nutrition* 78 (2003): 40–46.

22. Chamberlain, J., "The Possible Role of Long-Chain, Omega-3 Fatty Acids in Human Brain Phylogeny," *Perspectives in Biology and Medicine* 39, no. 3 (1996): 436–445; Broadhurst, C., S. Cunnane, et al., "Rift Valley Lake Fish and Shellfish Provided Brain-Specific Nutrition for Early Homo," *British Journal of Nutrition* 79, no. 1 (1998): 3–21.

23. Stoll, A. L., and C. A. Locke, "Omega-3 Fatty Acids in Mood Disorders: A Review of Neurobiologic and Clinical Applications," *Natural Medications for Psychiatric Disorders: Considering the Alternatives,*

D. Mischoulon and J. Rosenbaum (Philadelphia: Lippincott Williams & Wilkins, 2002), 13–34.

24. I borrowed this graphic metaphor from Jeanette Settle. Settle, J. E., "Diet and Essential Fatty Acids," *Handbook of Complementary and Alternative Therapies in Mental Health*, S. Shannon (San Diego: Academic Press, 2001) 93–113.

25. Weissman, M. W., R. Bland, et al., "Cross-National Epidemiology of Major Depression and Bipolar Disorder," *Journal of the American Medical Association* 276 (1996): 293–296; Hibbeln, J. (1998).

26. Stordy, B., and M. Nichol, *The LCP Solution: The Remarkable Nutritional Treatment for ADHD, Dyslexia, and Dyspraxia* (New York: Ballantine Books, 2000).

27. Klerman, G. L., and M. M. Weissman, "Increasing Rates of Depression," *Journal of the American Medical Association* 261, no. 15 (1989): 2229–2235.

28. Endres, S., R. Ghorbani, et al., "The Effect of Dietary Supplementation with n-3 Polyunsaturated Fatty Acids on the Synthesis of Interleukin-1 and Tumor Necrosis Factor by Mononuclear Cells," *New England Journal of Medicine* 320, no. 5 (1989): 265–271; Simopoulos, A.,"Omega-3 Fatty Acids in Inflammation and Autoimmune Diseases," *Journal of the American College of Nutrition* 21, no. 6 (2002): 495–505; Stoll, A. L., and C. A. Locke, "Omega-3 Fatty Acids in Mood Disorders: A Review of Neurobiologic and Clinical Applications," *Natural Medications for Psychiatric Disorders: Considering the Alternatives*, D. Mischoulon and J. Rosenbaum (Philadelphia: Lippincott Williams & Wilkins, 2002), 13–34.

29. Rudin, D. O., "The Dominant Diseases of Modernized Societies as Omega-3 Essential Fatty Acid Deficiency Syndrome," *Medical Hypotheses* 8 (1982): 17–47; Simopoulos, A. P., and J. Robinson, *The Omega Diet* (New York: Harper Collins, 1998).

30. Liu, K., J. Stamler, et al., "Dietary Lipids, Sugar, Fiber, and Mortality from Coronary Heart Disease—Bivariate Analysis of International Data," *Atherosclerosis* 2 (1998): 221–227.

31. Weissman, M. W., R. Bland, et al., "Cross-National Epidemiology of Major Depression and Bipolar Disorder," *Journal of the American Medical Association* 276 (1996): 293–296.

32. De Lorgeril, M., S. Renaud, et al., "Mediterranean Alpha-Linolenic Acid Rich Diet in Secondary Prevention of Coronary Heart Disease," *The Lancet* 343 (1994): 1454–1459.

33. Christensen, J. H., and E. B. Schmidt, "N-3 Fatty Acids and the Risk of Sudden Cardiac Death," *Lipids* 36 (2001): S115–118; Leaf, A., "Electrophysiologic Basis for the Antiarrhythmic and Anticonvulsant Effects of Omega-3 Polyunsaturated Fatty Acids," *World Review of Nutrition & Dietetics* 88 (2001): 72–78; Brouwer, I. A., P. L. Zock, et al., "Association Between n-3 Fatty Acid Status in Blood and Electrocardiographic Predictors of Arrhythmia Risk in Healthy Volunteers," *American Journal of Cardiology* 89, no. 5 (2002): 629–631.

34. Smith, R. S., "The Macrophage Theory of Depression," *Medical Hypotheses* 35 (1991): 298–306; Maes, M., and R. S. Smith, "Fatty Acids, Cytokines, and Major Depression," *Biological Psychiatry* 43 (1998): 313–314.

35. Crawford, M. A., "Fatty-Acid Ratios in Free-Living and Domestic Animals," *The Lancet* (1968): 1329–1333; Crawford, M. A., M. M. Gale, et al., "The Polyenoic Acids and Their Elongation Products in the Muscle Tissue of Phacochoerus Aethiopicus: a Re-Evaluation of Animal Fat," *Journal of Biochemistry* 114 (1969): 68P; Crawford, M. A., M. M. Gale, et al., "Linoleic Acid and Linolenic Acid Elongation Products in the Muscle Tissue of Syncerus caffer and Other Ruminant Species," *Journal of Biochemistry* 115 (1969): 25–27.

36. Simopoulos, A. P., and N. Salem, "Omega-3 Fatty Acids in Eggs from Range-Fed Greek Chickens," *New England Journal of Medicine* (1989): 1412.

37. Renaud, S., M. Ciavatti, et al., "Protective Effects of Dietary Calcium and Magnesium on Platelet Function and Atherosclerosis in Rabbits Fed Saturated Fat," *Atherosclerosis* 47 (1983): 189–198.

38. Simopoulos, A. P., and J. Robinson, *The Omega Diet* (1998), op. cit.

39. Weill, P., et al., "Enriching Diets with Omega-3 Fatty Acid: Impact of Various Sources," *Nutrition, Metabolism, and Cardiovascular Diseases* (in press).

40. Marangell, L., J. Martinez, et al., "A Double-Blind, Placebo-Controlled Study of the Omega-3 Fatty Acid Docosahexaenoic Acid (DHA) in the Treatment of Major Depression," *American Journal of Psychiatry* 160, no. 5 (2003): 996–998.

41. Whereas daily vitamins have long been scorned by conventional medicine, they have recently made a significant comeback when a panel of experts published their conclusions in the *Journal of the American Medical Association*. After reviewing a large number of studies, the preeminent authors of this article were forced to acknowledge that daily vitamin intake (particularly vitamins B, E, C, and D) reduces the risk for a whole array of chronic illnesses and of serious diseases. Fletcher, R. H., and K. M. Fairfield, "Vitamins for Chronic Disease Prevention in Adults: Clinical Applications," *Journal of the American Medical Association* 287, no. 23 (2002): 3127–3129.

42. Stoll, A. L., *The Omega-3 Connection* (New York: Simon & Schuster, 2001).

43. Baillie, R. A., R. Takada, et al., "Coordinate Induction of Peroxisomal Acyl-Coa Oxidase and UCP-3 by Dietary Fish Oil: A Mechanism for Decreased Body Fat Deposition," *Prostaglandins, Leukotrienes & Essential Fatty Acids* 60, no. 5–6 (1999): 351–356.

44. Kris-Etherton, P. M., W. S. Harris, et al., "AHA Scientific Statement: Fish Consumption, Fish Oil, Omega-3 Fatty Acids, and Cardiovascular Disease," *Circulation* 106 (2002): 2747–2757.

Chapter 10: Prozac or Puma?

1. McDonald, D. G., and J. A. Hogdon, *The Psychological Effects of Aerobic Fitness Training: Research and Theory* (New York: Springer-Verlag, 1991); Long, B. C., and R. van Stavel, "Effects of Exercise Training on

Anxiety. A Meta-Analysis," *Journal of Applied Sport Psychology* 7 (1995): 167–189.

2. DiLorenzo, T. M., E. P. Bargman, et al., "Long-Term Effects of Aerobic Exercise on Psychological Outcomes," *Preventive Medicine* 28, no. 1 (1999): 75–85.

3. Kasch, F., "The Effects of Exercise on the Aging Process," *The Physician and Sports Medicine* 4 (1976): 64–68; Palone, A. M., R. R. Lewis, et al., "Results of Two Years of Exercise Training in Middle-Aged Men," *The Physician and Sports Medicine* 4 (1976): 72–77.

4. LaPerrière, A., M. H. Antoni, et al., "Exercise Intervention Attenuates Emotional Distress and Natural Killer Cell Decrements Following Notification of Positive Serologic Status of HIV-1," *Biofeedback and Self-Regulation* 15 (1990): 229–242.

5. Greist, J. H., M. H. Klein, et al., "Running as Treatment for Depression," *Comprehensive Psychiatry* 20, no. 1 (1979): 41–54.

6. Beck, A., *Depression: Clinical, Experimental and Theoretical Aspects* (New York: Harper & Row, 1967); Beck, A., *Cognitive Therapy and the Emotional Disorders* (New York: International Universities Press, 1976); Burns, D. D., *The New Mood Therapy* (1999).

7. Babyak, M., J. A. Blumenthal, et al., "Exercise Treatment for Major Depression: Maintenance and Therapeutic Benefit at 10 Months," *Psychosomatic Medicine* 62, no. 5 (2000): 633–638.

8. Blumenthal, J., M. Babyak, et al., "Effects of Exercise Training on Older Patients with Major Depression," *Archives of Internal Medicine* 159 (1999): 2349–2356.

9. Paffenbarger, R. S., I. M. Lee, et al., "Physical Activity and Personal Characteristics Associated with Depression and Suicide in American College Men," *Acta Psychiatrica Scandinavica* 377 (1994): 16–22.

10. Wise, S. P., and M. Herkenham, "Opiate Receptor Distribution in the Cerebral Cortex of the Rhesus Monkey," *Science* 218 (1982): 387–389.

11. Panksepp, J., M. Siviy, et al., "Brain Opioids and Social Emotions," *The Psychobiology of Attachment and Separation*, M. Reite and T. Field (New York: Academic Press, 1985).

12. Thoren, P., J. S. Floras, et al., "Endorphins and Exercise: Physiological Mechanisms and Clinical Implications," *Medicine & Science in Sports & Exercise* 22, no. 4 (1990): 417–428; Sher, L., "Exercise, Well-Being, and Endogenous Molecules of Mood," *The Lancet* 348, no. 9025 (1996): 477.

13. Jonsdottir, I. H., P. Hoffmann, et al., "Physical Exercise, Endogenous Opioids and Immune Function," *Acta Physiologica Scandinavica* 640, suppl.(1997): 47–50.

14. Furlan, R., D. Piazza, et al., "Early and Late Effects of Exercise and Athletic Training on Neural Mechanisms Controlling Heart Rate," *Cardiovascular Research* 27 (1993): 482–488.

15. George, M., Z. Nahas, et al., "Vagus Nerve Stimulation Therapy: A Research Update," *Neurology* 59, no. 6, suppl. 4 (2002): S56–61.

16. Lawlor, D., and S. Hopker, "The Effectiveness of Exercise as an Intervention in the Management of Depression: Systematic Review and Meta-Regression Analysis of Randomised Controlled Trials," *British Medical Journal* 322, no. 7289 (2001): 763–767.

Chapter 11: Love Is a Biological Need

1. Observatoire National des Prescriptions et Consommations des Medicaments. *Etude de la Prescription et de la Consommation des antidepresseurs en Ambulatoire*. Paris, Agence du Médicament—Directions des Etudes et de l'Information Pharmaco-Economiques (1998).

2. Gupta, S., "If everyone were on Prozac . . ." *Time* 81 (January 20, 2003).

3. Hirigoyen, M.-F., *Stalking the Soul: On Emotional Abuse and the Erosion of Identity* (Helen Marx Books, 2000).

4. The cingular cortex is the oldest and the most "primitive" region of the neocortex, whose tissue is closer to that of the emotional brain than to that of the neocortex. Mesulam, M. M., *Principles of Behavioral Neurology* (Philadelphia: F. A. Davis, 1985).

5. Schanberg, S., "Genetic Basis for Touch Effects," *Touch in Early Development*, T. Field (Hillsdale, NJ: Erlbaum, 1994): 67–80. The remarkable research of Dr. Tiffany Field on growth of preterm babies preceded the explanation of Dr. Schanberg by several years. Field, T., S. M. Schanberg, et al., "Tactile/Kinesthetic Stimulation Effects on Preterm Neonates," *Pediatrics* 77 (1986): 654–658.

6. Spitz, R., "Hospitalism: An Inquiry into the Genesis of Psychiatric Conditions in Early Childhood," *Psychoanalytic Study of the Child* I (1945): 53–74.

7. Hubel, D., "The Visual Cortex of Normal and Deprived Monkeys," *American Scientist* 67, no. 5 (1979): 532–543.

8. Chugani, H. T., M. E. Behen, et al., "Local Brain Functional Activity Following Early Deprivation: A Study of Postinstitutionalized Romanian Orphans," *Neuroimage* 14, no. 6 (2001): 1290–1301.

9. Hofer, M. A., "Early Social Relationships: A Psychobiologist's View," *Child Development* 58 (1987): 633–647. I wish to thank the remarkable book of Tom Lewis, Fari Amini, and Richard Lannon, *A General Theory of Love*, for bringing this experiment to my attention.

10. Katz, L. F., and J. M. Gottman, "Buffering Children from Marital Conflict and Dissolution," *Journal of Clinical Child Psychology* 26 (1997): 157–171.

11. Murray Parkes, C., B. Benjamin, et al., "Broken Heart: A Statistical Study of Increased Mortality among Widowers," *British Medical Journal* 646 (1969): 740–743.

12. Medalie, J. H., and U. Goldbourt, "Angina Pectoris among 10,000 men. II. Psychosocial and Other Risk Factors as Evidenced by a Multivariate Analysis of a Five Year Incidence Study," *American Journal of Medicine* 60, no. 6 (1976): 910–921.

13. Medalie, J. H., K. C. Stange, et al., "The Importance of Biopsychosocial Factors in the Development of Duodenal Ulcer in a Cohort of Middle-Aged Men," *American Journal of Epidemiology* 136, no. 10 (1992): 1280–1287.

14. Reynolds, P., P. T. Boyd, et al., "The Relationship Between Social Ties and Survival among Black and White Breast Cancer Patients. National Cancer Institute Black/White Cancer Survival Study Group," *Cancer Epidemiology, Biomarkers & Prevention* 3, no. 3 (1994): 253–259.

15. Levenson, R., L. L. Carstensen, et al., "Long-Term Marriage: Age, Gender, and Satisfaction," *Psychology and Aging* 8, no. 2 (1993): 301–313.

16. Graham, C. A., and W. C. McGrew, "Menstrual Synchrony in Female Undergraduates Living on a Coeducational Campus," *Psychoneuroendocrinology* 5 (1980): 245–252.

17. Lewis, T., F. Amini, et al., *A General Theory of Love* (New York: Random House, 2000).

18. Friedman, E., and S. A. Thomas, "Pet Ownership, Social Support, and One-Year Survival after Acute Myocardial Infarction in the Cardiac Arrhythmia Suppression Trial (CAST)," *American Journal of Cardiology* 76 (1995): 1213–1217.

19. Siegel, J. M., "Stressful Life Events and Use of Physician Services among the Elderly: The Moderating Influence of Pet Ownership," *Journal of Personal and Social Psychology* 58 (1990): 1081–1086.

20. Rodin, J., Langer, E. J., "Long-Term Effects of a Control-Relevant Intervention with the Institutionalized Aged," *Journal of Personality and Social Psychology* 35 (1977): 897–902.

21. Siegel, J. M., F. J. Angulo, et al., "AIDS Diagnosis and Depression in the Multicenter AIDS Cohort Study: The Ameliorating Impact of Pet Ownership," *AIDS Care* 11 (1999): 157–169.

22. Allen, K., and J. Blascovich, "The Value of Service Dogs for People with Severe Ambulatory Disabilities: A Randomized Controlled Trial," *Journal of the American Medical Association* 275 (1996): 1001–1006.

23. Lockwood, R., "The Influence of Animals on Social Perception," *New Perspectives on Our Lives with Companion Animals*, vol. 8, A. H. Katcher and A. M. Beck (Philadelphia: University of Pennsylvania Press, 1983): 64–71.

24. Allen, K., B. E. Shykoff, et al., "Pet Ownership, but Not ACE Inhibitor Therapy, Blunts Home Blood Pressure Responses to Mental Stress," *Hypertension* 38 (2001): 815–820.

25. Allen, K., and J. L. Izzo, "Social Support and Resting Blood Pressure among Young and Elderly Women: The Moderating Role of Pet Ownership" (in submission).

26. Simon, S., "Sarajevo Pets," Weekend Edition Saturday with Scott Simon, Washington, National Public Radio (1993).

Chapter 12: Enchancing Emotional Communication

1. Hocker, J. L., and W. W. Wilmot, *Interpersonal Conflict* (Dubuque, IA: William C. Brown, 1991).

2. Chang, P. P., D. E. Ford, et al., "Anger in Young Men and Subsequent Premature Cardiovascular Disease: The Precursors Study," *Archives of Internal Medicine* 162 (2002): 901–906.

3. Gottman, J., *Why Marriages Succeed or Fail* (New York: Simon & Schuster, 1994); Gottman, J., and N. Silver, *The Seven Principles for Making Marriage Work* (New York:Random House, 1994).

4. Levenson, R., L. L. Carstensen, et al., "Long-term marriage: Age, gender, and satisfaction," *Psychology and Aging* no. 8 (1993): 301–313.

5. Gottman, J., *What Predicts Divorce* (Mahwaw, NJ: Lawrence Erlbaum Associates, 1994): 84, cited in Goleman, D., *Emotional Intelligence* (New York: Bantam Books, 1995): 135.

6. Rosenberg, M. D., *Non-violent Communication* (Puddle Dancer Press, 1999).

7. Harvey, O. J., *Conceptual Systems and Personality Organization* (New York: Harper & Row, 1961), cited in Rosenberg, M. D., op. cit.

Chapter 13: Listening with the Heart

1. Stuart, M. R., and J. A. Lieberman, *The Fifteen Minute Hour: Applied Psychotherapy for the Primary Care Physican* (Westport, Conn.: Prager, 1993).

2. Coulehan, J. L., and M. R. Block, *The Medical Interview: Mastering Skills for Clinical Practice*, 4th ed. (F.A. Davis Company, 2000).

3. Thank you to my friend and colleague Jo Devlin, M.S.W., for teaching me this metaphor about the benefits of briefly sharing the patient's burden of pain.

Chapter 14: The Larger Connection

1. Cherlin, *Marriage, Divorce and Remarriage* (Cambridge: Harvard University Press, 1992).

2. Klerman, G. L., and M. M. Weissman, "Increasing Rates of Depression," *Journal of the American Medical Association* 261, no. 15 (1989): 2229–2235.

3. Wilson, E. O., *Sociobiology: The New Synthesis*, 25th anniversary ed. (Cambridge: Harvard University Press, 2000).

4. Walsh, R., *Essential Spirituality: The Seven Central Practices to Awaken Heart and Mind* (New York: John Wiley & Sons, 1999).

5. Damasio, A., *Looking for Spinoza: Joy, Sorrow and the Feeling Brain* (San Diego: Harcourt, 2003).

6. Myers, D. G., and E. Diener, "The pursuit of happiness," *Scientific American* 274 (1996): 70–72; Argyle, M., *The Psychology of Happiness*, 20th ed. (New York: Routledge, 2001).

7. Durkheim, E., *Le Suicide. Une étude sociologique* (Paris: Alcan, 1897).

8. Zuckerman, D. M., S. V. Kasl, et al., "Psychosocial Predictors of Mortality among the Elderly Poor," *American Journal of Cardiology* 119 (1984): 410–423.

9. House, J. S., K. R. Landis, et al., "Social Relationships and Health," *Science* 241 (1988): 540–545.

10. Frankl, V. E., *Man's Search for Meaning: An Introduction to Logotherapy* (New York: 1976).

11. Mother Teresa quoted in Walsh, R. (1999), op. cit.

12. Abraham Maslow quoted in Walsh, R. (1999), op. cit.

13. McCraty, R., M. Atkinson, et al., "The Effects of Emotions on Short-Term Power Spectrum Analysis and Heart Rate Variability," *American Journal of Cardiology* 76, no. 14 (1995): 1089–1093.

Chapter 15: Getting Started

1. Aristotle, *Nichomacean Ethics*.

2. I wish to thank Dr. Scott Shannon, of the American Association of Holistic Medicine, for having pointed out the connection between Aristotle, Jung, and Maslow—across a span of 2,500 years—in the introduction to his book on natural methods in mental health. Shannon, S., *Integration and Holism. Handbook of Complementary and Alternative Therapies in Mental Health*, S. Shannon, ed. (San Diego: Academic Press, 2001): 21–42.

3. McCraty, R., M. Atkinson, et al., "The Effects of Emotions on Short-Term Power Spectrum Analysis and Heart Rate Variability," *American Journal of Cardiology* 76, no. 14 (1995): 1089–1093; Wilson, D., S. M. Silver, et al.,"Eye Movement Desensitization and Reprocessing: Effectiveness and Autonomic Correlates," *Journal of Behavior Therapy and Experimental Psychiatry* 27 (1996): 219–229; Rechlin, T., M. Weis, et al., "Does Bright-Light Therapy Influence Autonomic Heart-Rate Parameters?" *Journal of Affective Disorders* 34, no. 2 (1995): 131–137; Haker, E., H. Egekvist, et al.,"Effect of Sensory Stimulation (Acupuncture) on Sympathetic and Parasympathetic Activities in Healthy Subjects," *Journal of the Autonomic Nervous System* 79, no.1 (2000): 52–59; Christensen, J. H., M. S. Christensen, et al., "Heart Rate Variability and Fatty Acid Content of Blood Cell Membranes: A Dose-Response Study with n-3 Fatty Acids," *American Journal of*

Clinical Nutrition 70 (1999): 331–337; Furlan, R., D. Piazza, et al., "Early and Late Effects of Exercise and Athletic Training on Neural Mechanisms Controlling Heart Rate," *Cardiovascular Research* 27 (1993): 482–488; Porges, S. W., J. A. Doussard-Roosevelt, et al., "Vagal Tone and the Physiological Regulation of Emotion," *Monographs of the Society for Research in Child Development* 59, no. 2–3 (1994): 167–186, 250–283.

4. Keller, M., J. McCullough, et al., "A Comparison of Nefazodone, the Cognitive Behavioral-Analysis System of Psychotherapy, and Their Combination for the Treatment of Chronic Depression," *New England Journal of Medicine* 342 (2000): 1462–1470.

5. Ehlers, C., E. Frank, et al.,"Social Zeitgebers and Biological Rhythms. A Unified Approach to Understanding the Etiology of Depression," *Archives of General Psychiatry* 45, no. 10 (1988): 948–952.

Index

Underscored page references indicate boxed text. **Boldface** references indicate illustrations. Page references followed by the letter "n" indicate footnotes.

A

Acupuncture
  author's introductions to, 109–11
  author's personal encounter with, 113–15
  for depression, 110, 111
    patient story of, 117–18
  effectiveness of, 112–13
  effects of
    on autonomic nervous system, 120–21
    on emotional brain, 119–20
  finding practitioner of, 228
  influencing qi, 110, 120–21
  insurance coverage of, 246
  mechanisms of action of, 118–21
  meridians in, 115
  for pain relief, 119–20, 120n, 227–28
  placebo effect and, 111, 112
  for preoperative anxiety, 118
  resources on, 246–47
  scientific experiment on, 115–17
  when to use, 227–28
  yin and yang in, 116–17
Acute medical conditions, modern treatment of, 217–18
Adaptive information processing system, EMDR and, 78, 79, 82, 89
Affect, in BATHE technique for listening, 196
Aggressive behavior
  for handling conflict, 177
  situations calling for, 191
Altruism, source of, 211
Amini, Fari, 169
Amygdala, **10**, 22
Anecdotes, caution about, 132–33
Anti-anxiety medications, reliance on, for self-soothing, 220

Antibiotics, 217
Antidepressants
  for fibromyalgia, 103
  placebo effect and, 95, 111
  prevalence of, 8, 162–63
  relapse after discontinuing, 9
  reliance on, for self-soothing,
    220
Antipsychotic medications,
    emotional apathy from, 14
Anxiety
  effect of exercise on, 147–48
  preoperative, acupuncture for,
    118
Anxiety attacks, 28–29
  autonomic nervous system and,
    156
  heart accelerations in, 40
  patient stories of, 36–37,
    145–47, 201
Aristotle, 216
Arrhythmias, 40
Autocompletion, 216
Autonomic nervous system
  balance provided by, 38
  effect of acupuncture on, 120–21
  effect of exercise on, 156, 157
  function of, 37–38
Autonomy, disadvantages of, 209
Avery, David, 103–4

B

Baby blues. *See* Depression,
    postpartum
Background information, in BATHE
    technique for listening, 195

BATHE technique for listening,
    195–200, 224
  developers of, 194–95
Beck, Aaron, 151
Bernard, Claude, 23
Biofeedback, for achieving cardiac
    coherence, 56, 221–22
Biological clock
  factors affecting, 101–2
  resetting, with dawn simulation,
    104–7, 226–27
Biological psychiatry, 8–9
Bipolar disorder
  lithium for, 93
  omega-3 fatty acids for, 129
  patient story of, 126–29
Blood pressure, effect of cardiac
    coherence on, 59
Brain
  cognitive, 21, 22
    in competition vs. harmony
      with emotional brain, 26–27
    controlling emotions, 29–31
  emotional (limbic), 21–22
    acupuncture affecting, 119–20
    and body, relationship with,
      24–25
    in competition vs. harmony
      with cognitive brain, 26–27
    cravings of, 232
    disconnecting from cognitive
      brain in trauma, 72, 74–75
    disorders associated with, 11
    functions of, 11, 22–24, 27
    and heart, relationship
      between, 34, 37, 40, 54–55
    limbic communication
      affecting, 164

self-healing mechanisms of, 11
   short-circuiting of, 27–29
   social relations and, 159
   structure of, 10–11, **10**, 22, 23
evolution of, 20, 22
neocortex, 22, 25–26
nutrition affecting, 124–25, 143
scars in
   indelibility of, 73
   patient story of, 73–74
   from trauma, 70–71
Brazelton, T. Berry, 18
Breathing, in cardiac coherence
      training, 53
Broca, Paul, 22

C

Cade, John F. J., 93n
Camus, Albert, 210–11, 231–32
Cancer, depression as symptom of,
   137
Cannon, Walter B., 183
Cardiovascular disease
   depression and, 135–36
   omega-3 fatty acids for, 136
Case studies, sources of, 2
Chaos, physiological, 42–43, **42**,
   45–46, 50, **57**
Cho, Zhang-Hee, 116
Chronic medical conditions, modern
      treatment of, 217–18
Chronic psychiatric conditions,
      treatment of
   nontraditional, 6–7
   synergistic, 218–19
   traditional, 6

Cod liver oil, as unreliable source
   of omega-3s, 142
Cognitive-behavior therapy,
   effectiveness of, 8
Cohen, Jonathan, 22
Coherence, cardiac
   from acupuncture, 120
   benefits from, 66
      emotional, 61
      physical, 58–61
      social, 61–62
   blocked access to, 67
   brain function and, **57**
   from connection with others,
      213
   emotional brain and, 54–55
   emotional communication and,
      206
   energy saved by, 47
   example of, 46
   exercise increasing, 156, 157
   in heart rate variability, 42–43,
      42, 45
   living in, examples of, 62–66
   physiology influenced by,
      46–47
   positive effects of, 48, 50
   from prayer, 56, 58
   resources on, 240–42
   software for, 41–43, 221–22
   for stress management, 48–49
   training method, 52–55, 221,
      222
      patient story of, 47–48
   when to use, 221
   from yoga, 56
Communication, emotional. *See*
      Emotional communication

Conflict
    appropriate responses to, 185–88
    for enriching relationships,
        223–24
    with STABEN approach,
        188–91, 192, 224
    behaviors for handling, 176–78,
        191–92
    chronic, between couples, 179–80
    inappropriate responses to,
        181–85
    management, resources on,
        248–50
Connection with others
    benefits of, 211–13
    guidelines for finding, 228–29
    as human drive, 211
    for meaning in life, 209
    patient story of, 209–10
Contempt, as obstacle to
        communication, 182–83
Cook, Frederick, 99–100
Counterattack, as obstacle to
        communication, 183–84
Couples, chronic conflict between,
        179–80
Cretan Diet, 224
Criticism, as obstacle to
        communication, 181–82
Csikszentmihalyi, Mihaly, 1,
        31–32, 152, 158
Cure, meaning of, 1

D

Dairy products, omega-3 fatty acids
        and, 140–41

Damasio, Antonio, 1, 21, 23, 26,
        30, 35n, 211, 232
Darwin, Charles, 20, 22, 32
Dawn simulation
    as alternative to alarm clock,
        104–5
    guidelines for, 226–27
    patient experience with, 105
    potential benefits of, 106–7
    for protecting REM sleep, 106
    resources on, 244–46
Depression
    acupuncture for, 110, 111
        patient story of, 117–18
    from alienation, 209
    as cancer symptom, 137
    cardiovascular disease and,
        135–36
    Eastern vs. Western view of, 110
    exercise for
        author's experience with,
            153–54
        maximizing benefits of,
            157–59
        patient story of, 148–51
        preventive effects of, 153
        runner's high from, 151–52
        studies on, 152–53
    incidence of
        increase in, 162
        in Western vs. Asian countries,
            135
    inflammation theory of,
        136–37
    after myocardial infarction
        patient story of, 51–52
        as predictor of death, 34
    nontraditional treatment of, 6

omega-3 fatty acids for
  patient story of, 129–32
  required dosage, 141
  studies on, 133–34
pets for reducing, 170–172
postpartum
  incidence of, in Western vs.
    Asian countries, 124
  omega-3 fatty acids and, 124
  patient story of, 123–24
winter
  dawn simulation for, 104–5
  light therapy for, 103–4
  symptoms of, 102
Digestive system, "small brain" of, 36
Divorce rate, 209
Doctors Without Borders/Médecins
  Sans Frontières, 5
Dolto, Françoise, 62
Dream sleep, 105–6
Drug use, illegal, for self-soothing,
  220
Durkheim, Emile, 211–12

E

EMDR. *See* Eye movement
    desensitization and
    reprocessing
Emotion(s)
  cardiac coherence and, 61
  danger from excessive control of,
    29–31
  expressing, in nonviolent
    communication, 186–87,
    190
  function of, 13, 23–24

negative, chaos from, 45
  as physical state, 35
  positive, coherence from, 45
  rationality and, 15
Emotional apathy, from mental
    illness, 13–14
Emotional brain. *See* Brain,
    emotional (limbic)
Emotional communication, 174
  for enriching relationships,
    223–24
  failure to teach, 200
  mastery of, 205–6
  nonviolent
    example of, 177–79
    principles of, 185–88
    STABEN approach to, 188–91,
      192, 224
  obstacles to, 180–81
    contempt, 182–83
    counterattack, 183–84
    criticism, 181–82
    stonewalling, 183, 184–85
  patient story of, 200–205
  resources on, 248–50
  in social relations, 164
Emotional flooding, 180, 189
Emotional intelligence
  cultivation of, 32
  definition of, 15
  equilibrium and, 31
  success and, 16, 19
Emotional mastery, key to, 37
Emotional neglect, effects of, 167
Emotional quotient (EQ)
  aptitudes related to, 16–17,
    18–19
  poor, example of, 17–18

Emotional short-circuiting, 27–29

Emotional states, difficulty identifying, 18–19

Emotional violence
 effects of, 161–62
 examples of, 161
 overcoming, for reducing depression, 163

Empathy, in BATHE technique for listening, 199–200

Endorphins, exercise stimulating, 154–55

Energy
 loss, from chaos, 45–46
 saved, by coherence, 47

Eslinger, Paul, 30

Exercise
 for anxiety, 147–48
 for anxiety attacks, 146–47
 for depression
  author's experience with, 153–54
  patient story of, 148–51
  preventive effects of, 153
  runner's high from, 151–52
  studies on, 152–53
 endorphins stimulated by, 154–55
 as fun, 158–59
 group vs. individual, 158
 guidelines for, 225–26
 immune system stimulated by, 155
 maximizing benefits of, 157–59
 recommended amount of, 157–58

Exposure therapy, for removing fear response, 72–73

Eye movement desensitization and reprocessing (EMDR), 67
 adaptive information processing system and, 78, 79, 82, 89
 combined with other therapies, 95
 controversy and skepticism about, 75, 83, 91–92
 effectiveness of, 77–78, 91
  in children, 89–91
  recognition of, 94–95
 finding practitioner of, 222–23
 founder of, 75
 healing process of, 82–83, 222
 insurance coverage of, 223
 mechanism of, 93–94
 negative results of, 95, 97–98
 patient stories of, 76–77, 85–89, 97
 recovery from illness and, 89n
 resources on, 242–44

F

Facial expressions, contempt shown in, 183

Fatigue
 chronic, patient story of, 102–3
 mental, cardiac coherence reducing, 60–61

Fear response, exposure therapy for removing, 72–73

Feelings. *See also* Emotion(s)
 expressing, in nonviolent communication, 186–87, 190
 power of, 162

Fibromyalgia, 102–3

Fifteen Minute Hour, The (Stuart and Lieberman), 195n

Fight and flight, as response to attack, 183

Fish, omega-3 fatty acids in, 138, 138n, <u>139</u>

Fish oil supplements, 141–42, 225, 247–48

Flax, omega-3 fatty acids in, 138, 138n, <u>139</u>, 248

"Flow," state of, 32, 35
  from exercise, 152, 158

Frankl, Victor, 212

Freud, Sigmund, 20–21, 79, 96

G

Gage, Phineas, 30

General Theory of Love, A (Lewis et al.), 169

Goleman, Daniel, 1, 15, 19

Gottman, John, 179, 180, 181, 185, 189, 249

Gottman, Julie Schwartz, 249

Gratitude, heart's sensitivity to, 54

Greist, John, 148

Grief work, 79

Grievances, stating, without criticism, 181–82

H

Handling, in BATHE technique for listening, 198–99

Harmony, balance required for, 31–32

Heart
  communicating with, 55
  emotional brain and, 34, 37, 40
  hormones produced by, 36
  influencing whole body, 36
  "small brain" of, 36

Heart attack. *See* Myocardial infarction

Heart-brain system, 34, **39**
  effect of trauma on, 67
  harmony in, effects of, 34–35

Heart coherence. *See* Coherence, cardiac

Heart disease, stress and, 34

Heart failure, effect of cardiac coherence on, 58

Heart rate variability
  chaotic vs. coherent, 42–43, **42**
  computer measurement of, 41–43, 50, 55–56, 58
  effect of stress on, 41
  exercise increasing, 155–56
  as healthy state, 40
  loss of
    with aging, 43
    as danger sign, 40
    health problems from, 43–44
  omega-3 fatty acids and, 136
  patient story of, 44–45, 47–48

Hermann, Judith, 1

Hofer, Myron, 167

Homeostasis, 23

Hormone balance, effect of cardiac coherence on, 59

Horrobin, David, 141

Hubel, David, 166–67

Hugo, Victor, 184–85
Hui, Kathleen, 118–19
Human beings
    limbic communication among,
        164
    young, nurturing of, 163–64
Hypothalamus, function of, 100,
        101–2

I

Immune system
    cardiac coherence and, 59–60
    exercise stimulating, 155
    meditation and, 60n
Individuation, 216
Inflammation theory of depression,
        136–37
Inflammatory reactions, omega-6
        fatty acids and, 135
Intelligence
    definition of, 15
    emotional (*see* Emotional
        intelligence)
    types of, 16
Intelligence quotient (IQ)
    constancy of, 32
    success and, 15–16
IQ Test, 15
"I" statements, in nonviolent
        communication, 186–87

J

James, William, 35
Janet, Pierre, 96

Jogging
    for depression
        patient story of, 148–51
        vs. Zoloft treatment, 152
        runner's high from, 151–52
Judgment, avoiding, in nonviolent
        communication, 185–86
Jung, Carl, 16, 216

K

Kabat-Zinn, Jon, 60n
Karajan, Herbert von, effect of
        music on, 33–34
Kitchen Table Wisdom (Remen), 199n
Kramer, Peter, 9
Kübler-Ross, Elizabeth, 87

L

Lannon, Richard, 169
LaPerrière, Arthur, 148
LeDoux, Joseph, 1, 72, 73
Lewis, Tom, 1, 169
Lieberman, Joseph A., 194, 195,
        195n
Light
    artificial vs. natural, 100–101
    internal cycles trained by, 101
    mood and drives influenced by,
        100
        historical accounts of, 99–100
Light therapy
    with dawn simulation (*see* Dawn
        simulation)
    with light box, 103, 107

Limbic brain. *See* Brain, emotional
(limbic)
Limbic regulation, 169
Listening
    author's experience in teaching,
        193–94
    with BATHE technique,
        194–200, 224
Listening to Prozac (Kramer), 9
Lithium, early FDA resistance to,
    93, 93n
Looking for Spinoza (Damasio), 35n
Lorgeril, Michel de, 136
Love
    affecting adult physiology,
        168–69
    human drive for, 174
    mother, affecting newborn
        physiology, 167, 168
    physiology of, 163–64
    relationships, autonomic nervous
        system and, 38, 40
Love Lab of Seattle, 179–81
Luskin, Frederic, 58

M

Mammals
    autonomic nervous system in,
        38
    baby, vulnerability of, 163–64
    limbic communication among,
        164
Manic-depression. *See* Bipolar
    disorder
Man's Search for Meaning (Frankl),
    212

Marshall, Barry, 93n
Maslow, Abraham, 213, 216
McClelland, James, 5
Meats, omega-3 and omega-6 fatty
    acids in, 140
Medical breakthroughs, resistance
    to, 92–93
Medical treatment
    of acute vs. chronic conditions,
        217–18
    loss of synergy in, 217
Medications, for stress-related
    problems, 8, 9
Meditation
    for autonomic balance, 121
    immune function and, 60n
Melatonin production, 101n
Memories
    accessing, 81
    emotional, indelibility of, 73
    traumatic
        addressing, with EMDR (*see*
            Eye movement
            desensitization and
            reprocessing)
        locked in nervous system,
            80–81
        triggering of, patient story of,
            81–82
Mental illness, emotional apathy
    from, 13–14
Meridians, in acupuncture, 115
Morant, Soulié de, 109
Mother love, affecting newborn
    physiology, 167, 168
Mother Teresa, 212–13
Mourning and Melancholia (Freud),
    79

Myocardial infarction, depression
        after
    patient story of, 51–52
    as predictor of death, 34
Myth of Sisyphus, The (Camus),
        210–11

N

Natural killer cells, effect of
        exercise on, 148, 155, **156**
Needs, expressing, in nonviolent
        communication, 187, 191
Nemets, Boris, 133
Neocortex, 22, 25–26
Newborn physiology, mother love
        affecting, 167, **168**
Nolan, James, 43–44
Nonviolent assertive
        communication. *See*
        Emotional communication
Nonviolent Communication
        (Rosenberg), 185, 249
Nutrition
    for autonomic balance, 121
    effect of, on brain, 124–25, 143

O

Objectivity, in nonviolent
        communication, 185–86,
        190
Omega-3 Connection, The (Stoll), 129
Omega-3 fatty acids
    for bipolar disorder, 129
    for cardiovascular disease, 136

cautions about, 225
deficiency of
    linked to postpartum
        depression, 124
    mood changes from, 125
for depression, 131–32, 133–34
dosage of, for antidepressant
        effect, 141
in early humanoids, 134–35
effect of, on fetus and newborns,
        125–26
imbalance of, in Western diet,
        135
maximizing, in diet, 224–25
resources on, 247
sources of, 134, 138, <u>139</u>, 140–42
in supplement form, 141–42,
        225, 247–48
    side effects from, 142
    weight control with, 142
Omega-6 fatty acids
    in early humanoids, 134–35
    excess, inflammation from, 134,
        135
    food sources of, 134, 140
    imbalance of, in Western diet,
        135
Opium, effect of, on emotional
        brain, 154–55
Ornish, Dean, 1
Ost, Thomas, 117, 119
Overweight, stress and, 19

P

Pain relief, acupuncture for,
        119–20, 120n, 227–28

Panic attacks. *See* Anxiety attacks
Parasympathetic nervous system
  effect of exercise on, 156, 157
  function of, 38
  parental love affecting, 167–68
  strengthening, 216–17
Passive or passive aggressive
    behavior
  for handling conflict, 176
  situations calling for, 191
Pert, Candice, 121
Pets
  demonstrating drive to love,
    173–74
  health benefits from, 170–73
Piaget, Jean, 16
Placebo effect
  acupuncture and, 111
  antidepressants and, 95, 111
Pleasure, exercise stimulating, 154–55
Porges, Stephen, 38
Postpartum depression. *See*
    Depression, postpartum
Post-traumatic stress disorder
    (PTSD), 28
  in children, EMDR for treating,
    89–91
  ineffectiveness of treatments for,
    75
  psychiatric symptoms excluding,
    96
  scar in the brain from, 70–71
Prayer, cardiac coherence from, 56, 58
Prefrontal cortex
  functions of, 26
  stress affecting, 27–28
Premature infants, effect of touch
    on, 165–66

Psychoanalysis, decreasing
  popularity of, 8
Psychotherapy, cognitive-behavior
  therapy in, 8
Psychotropic medications, 9
Puri, Basant, 130–33

Q

Qi, 110, 120–21
Quirk, Greg, 73

R

Randomized placebo-controlled
  studies, 132–33
Relationship Cure, The (Gottman),
  179, 249
Remen, Rachel Naomi, 199n
REM sleep, 105–6
Renaud, Serge, 136, 140
Resilience
  characteristics of, 4
  development of, 79
Resistance to medical
  breakthroughs, 92–93
Resources
  on acupuncture, 246–47
  on cardiac coherence, 240–42
  on conflict management and
    emotional communication,
    248–50
  on dawn simulation, 244–46
  on EMDR, 242–44
  general, 239
  on omega-3 fatty acids, 247–48

Reston, James, 120n
Rosenberg, Marshall, 185, 186,
　　　187, 249
Runner's high, 151–52

S

Saint-Exupéry, Antoine de, 207
Sarcasm, as expression of contempt,
　　　182–83
Schonberg, Saul, 166
Seasonal affective disorder, 102. *See
　　　also* Depression, winter
Self-actualization, 213, 216
Self-centeredness, values of, 208
Semmelweis, Philippe, 92–93
Servan-Schreiber, David
　　background of, 4–6
　　inspiration of, 1–2
　　openness of, to nontraditional
　　　treatments, 6–7
Sexuality, cardiac coherence
　　　enhancing, 66
Shannon, Scott, 1
Shapiro, Francine, 75, 95n
Simon, Herbert, 5
Simopoulos, Artemis, 140–41
Sleep, dream, 105–6
Smile, as sign of harmony, 32
Social relations
　　cardiac coherence and, 61–62
　　emotional brain and, 159
　　limbic communication in, 164
　　physiology influenced by, 169
Sophrology, for treating
　　　depression, 6
Spinoza, 23

STABEN approach to conflict
　　　resolution, 188–91, 192,
　　　224
Stickgold, Robert, 93–94
Stoll, Andrew, 129, 141, 142, 248
Stonewalling, as obstacle to
　　　communication, 183,
　　　184–85
Stranger, The (Camus), 231–32
Stress
　　chronic, effects of, 49–50
　　heart rate variability and, 41
　　immune system and, 60
　　overweight and, 19
　　pets for reducing, 172
　　as risk factor for heart disease, 34
　　symptoms of, cardiac coherence
　　　reducing, 60–61
Stress disorders
　　increase in, 7–8
　　types of, 31
Stress management, coherence for,
　　　48–49
Stuart, Marian R., 194, 195, 195n
Success, factors determining,
　　　15–16, 19
Suicide (Durkheim), 211–12
Suicide, contributor to, 211–12
Sympathetic nervous system, 38,
　　　156
Synergy, in treatment of illness,
　　　216–17, 218–19

T

Tachycardia, 40
Talk therapy, decreasing use of, 8, 9

Tibetan medicine, 5–6
Touch, effects of, 165–67
Trauma
  effect of, on heart-mind system, 67
  inability to digest, 79
  memory of, locked in nervous system, 80–81
  patient stories of, 69–70, 79–80
  psychological disturbances from, 96
  scar in the brain from, 70–71
  "small t"
    digestion of, 78–79
    traces of pain from, 71–72, 96–97
Treatment methods for emotional problems
  nontraditional
    assumptions behind, 10–11
    mechanisms of, 7
    as presented in this book, 11–12
    for promoting harmony, 32
    synergistic, 218–19
    traditional, 6–7, 8
Treatment plan, principles in building
  acupuncture, 227–28
  addressing painful memories, 222–23
  dawn simulation, 226–27
  exercise, 225–26
  heart coherence, 219–22
  managing conflict and enriching relationships, 223–24
  maximizing omega-3s, 224–25
  seeking larger connection, 228–29
Trouble, in BATHE technique for listening, 196–97

U

Ulcer treatment, medical community resistance to, 93, 93n
University of Pittsburgh
  Center for Complementary Medicine, 219, 239
  psychiatry department of, 5
  Shadyside Hospital, natural treatment methods of, 9–10

V

Van Der Kolk, Bessel, 1, 80
Vegetable oils, omega-3 and omega-6 fatty acids in, 140
Vegetarian sources of omega-3 fatty acids, 138, 138n, 139, 140
Violence
  emotional (*see* Emotional violence)
  escalation of, from counterattacks, 183–84
  in response to stonewalling, 184
Vitamin E, taken with omega-3 supplements, 141–42
Volunteer work, benefits of, 211–12

W

Watkins, Alan, 52, 54, 240
Weil, Andrew, 1
Wiesel, Torsten, 166–67
Wind, Sand and Stars (Saint-Exupéry),
    selflessness illustrated in,
    207–8
Winter
    depression in (*see* Depression,
      winter)
    human drives affected by, 101–2
Winter, Dan, 52
Wortis, Joseph, 21

Y

Yin and yang, in acupuncture,
    116–17
Yoga, cardiac coherence from,
    56

Z

Zarcone, Vincent, 105–6
Zoloft, vs. jogging, for depression,
    152